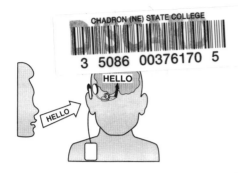

cochlear implants
and children:
a handbook for parents, teachers
and speech and hearing
professionals

D1520417

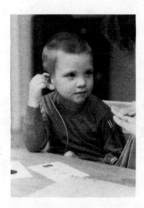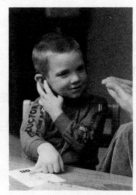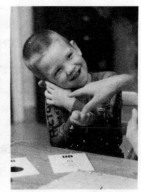

Becoming aware of sound can be an exciting process. This recently implanted, four-year-old child listens for a soft sound presented by his audiologist.
Photos by Warren Paris.

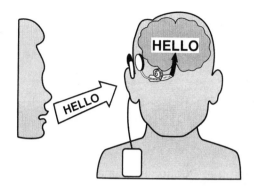

cochlear implants and children: a handbook for parents, teachers and speech and hearing professionals

nancy tye-murray, ph.d., editor-author

Alexander Graham Bell Association
for the Deaf
3417 Volta Place, N.W.
Washington, D.C. 20007

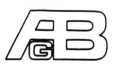

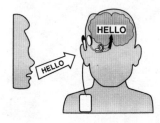

Library of Congress Cataloging in Publication Data

Tye-Murray, Nancy, Ph.D., Editor-Author
Cochlear Implants and Children:
A Handbook for Parents, Teachers and
Speech and Hearing Professionals

Library of Congress Catalog Card Number 91-076738
ISBN 0-88200-173-6
© 1992 Alexander Graham Bell Association for the Deaf
3417 Volta Place, N.W.
Washington, D.C. 20007

Printed in the United States of America

10   9   8   7   6   5   4   3   2   1

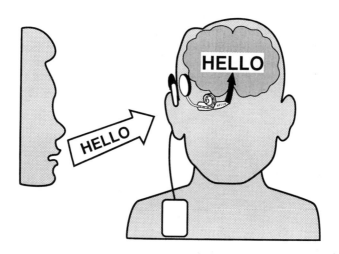

acknowledgments

We wish to acknowledge support by the National Institutes of Health grant DC00242; for the grant RR59 from the General Clinical Research Centers Program, Division of Research Resources, NIH; and for the support from a grant from the Lions Clubs of Iowa. To Jim Heller for his review of Appendix 2-1; to Mary Lowder and Danielle Kelsay for their comments and suggestions throughout the book; to Marla Ross for preparing the manuscript; to Ruben Barreras for photographing the figures; and to Tim Brandau for providing Figure 1-7. (p. 21), we express our warm appreciation.

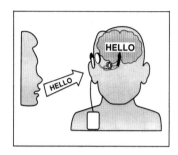

foreword

The cochlear implant has come of age as a rehabilitation tool for adults with no usable hearing. Implantation is no longer considered an experimental procedure, and the performance of many adult users has been remarkable.

Adults who have had normal hearing while acquiring speech and language seem to adapt to the electrical signal provided by the implant readily. In fact, they often reach their maximum listening potential within the first nine months of use. Adults usually can hear many environmental sounds and most can respond to normal levels of conversational speech. Many can understand speech well enough to conduct limited telephone conversations.

There is a wide variety of performance amongst adult users. Some cannot understand speech without lipreading while others can understand 90 percent of words spoken auditorily. As yet, we have not discovered why this variability exists. It does not appear to be strongly related to an implant user's age, intelligence, or cause of deafness.

The use of cochlear implants in profoundly deaf children is in its beginning stages. There are still many unanswered questions, such as: a) who is a good candidate, b) what is the optimal age to implant a child, c) how well will children hear, and d) what kind of learning curve will they demonstrate in developing auditory skills.

To date, results with children who have had limited hearing prior to receiving an implant have been encouraging, but differ greatly from those of the adult population. Their rate of learning to hear is much slower. Newly implanted children often do not react to sound initially. Developing sound awareness and learning to associate sound with speech takes time, just as it does in a normal hearing newborn. Some children who have been implanted two or three years are beginning to show marked speech recognition abilities. Perhaps in time they will perform as well as, or even better than, adult users, but only time will tell. What *is* encouraging is that implanted children have so much more potential for developing speech and the English language than they did without an implant. Age of implantation, parental support, and the type and amount of aural rehabilitation will likely influence the child's eventual functioning, but the interactions of these variables are not yet known.

We have entered upon a very exciting time in aural rehabilitation. This book will doubtlessly be reedited many times as the technology of cochlear implants develops. It provides a valuable resource to parents, teachers, and speech and hearing professionals who work with implanted children.

Mary Lowder, M.A. CCC-A
Cochlear Implant Audiologist
Iowa City, IA

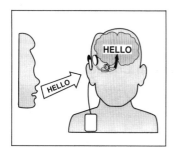

contents

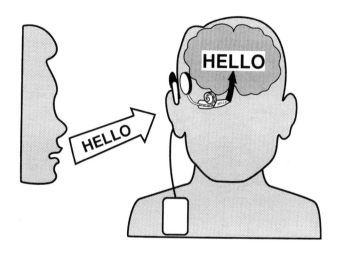

contributors

Holly Fryauf-Bertschy, M.A.
Karen Iler Kirk, Ph.D.
Nancy Tye-Murray, Ph.D.
Richard S. Tyler, Ph.D.

All contributors are affiliated with the Department of Otolaryngology—Head and Neck Surgery, University of Iowa Hospitals and Clinics, Iowa City, Iowa 52242

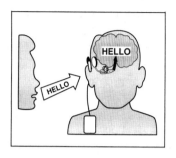

preface

The advent of cochlear implants initiates an exciting and challenging chapter in the history of the deaf community. Profoundly deaf children now have the potential to hear some speech and environmental sounds that they never would have heard otherwise. This book concerns the child who has either received a cochlear implant, or who is about to receive one. It was written for parents and teachers of cochlear implant recipients, and for speech and hearing professionals who work with implanted children or who are interested in learning about them.

The book applies to multichannel cochlear implant designs. The chapters pertaining to speech perception training and communication therapy are also relevant to moderately and severely hearing-impaired children who use hearing aids, since many of these children have listening skills similar to those of implanted children.

Chapters 1 and 2 describe the cochlear implant, how to maintain the device, and techniques for helping the child adjust to the implant in the home and school. Chapter 3 describes audiological measures used to assess auditory skills, and patient variables that influence performance. Communication modes and strategies for successfully conversing with an implanted child are considered in Chapter 4. Chapter 5 presents guidelines for developing the child's speech perception skills. A comprehensive auditory training and speechreading training program are presented in Chapters 6 and 7, respectively, along with specific lesson objectives and training procedures. Finally, Chapter 8 presents guidelines for communication therapy. It includes a large number of figures, which can be photocopied and used for teaching purposes.

The strength of this book lies in the contributing authors' clinical experience, and their familiarity with current research about cochlear implants and aural rehabilitation. The authors are part of a National Institutes of Health cochlear implant grant awarded to the University of Iowa. Collectively, the authors are experienced in adjusting and maintaining the cochlear implants of children and adults who have been implanted at the University of Iowa Hospitals and Clinics. They follow the implant recipients' audiological performance over time and provide them with aural rehabilitation and communication therapy. They also conduct an active research program. Two other individuals who are a part of the Iowa cochlear implant program, Mary Lowder and Danielle Kelsay, have contributed their ideas and suggestions, even though they are not listed as authors. Readers who are new to the field of cochlear implants and those who are knowledgeable should find this book interesting and helpful.

For the sake of clarity, male pronouns are used to refer to an implanted child. Female pronouns are used to refer to a parent, teacher, or speech and hearing professional. No gender stereotyping is intended by this practice.

The reader is asked to accept three propositions about cochlear implant use by children. First, implanted children vary greatly in their listening and speaking abilities. Regardless of how well the child performs with his device, parents and teachers should view their child as a successful individual. Secondly, parents should accept a primary role in helping their child adjust to the implant. They must assume responsibility for maintaining the implant device, for ensuring that the child is wearing it properly, and assuring that auditory speech stimulation occurs in both the home and school. Finally, the implanted child needs to develop a positive self image and a sense of belonging to his world. He should have ample opportunity to develop friendships with hearing and hearing-impaired children, and opportunity to socialize with other cochlear implant users.

Nancy Tye-Murray, Ph.D.
University of Iowa Hospitals and Clinics
Iowa City, IA

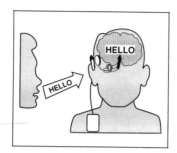

Phonetic Symbols for Sounds of General American English

Consonants	Vowels and diphthongs
/m/ me	/i/ bead
/w/ we	/ɪ/ bit
/b/ bee	/ɛ/ bed
/v/ van	/æ/ bad
/p/ pea	/a/ boss
/f/ fee	/ɔ/ ball
/ð/ that	/ʊ/ book
/θ/ thing	/ʌ/ bun
/n/ knee	/3˞/ bird
/l/ leap	/aɪ/ bite
/d/ deal	/oɪ/ boy
/z/ zeal	/u/ boot
/t/ tea	/e/ bait
/s/ sea	/o/ boat
/tʃ/ cheese	
/j/ yeast	
/r/ read	
/ʃ/ sheep	
/g/ geese	
/k/ key	
/h/ he	

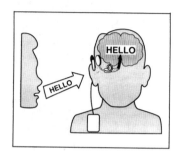

1

getting started at home
holly fryauf-bertschy, m.a.

Helping the newly implanted child learn to adjust to his hearing abilities can be exciting and challenging. Parents play the most significant role in helping the child accept and optimally use the cochlear implant. This chapter considers the implanted child who is ready to wear the external hardware and begin the process of learning to hear. The parts of the implant system are reviewed and suggestions for orienting the child to the device are offered.

components of the implant

The surgically implanted portion of a cochlear implant system consists of a receiver, an internal magnet, and an electrode array. During surgery, a small space is made in the child's mastoid bone behind his ear to accommodate the internal magnet and receiver. The electrode array is placed in direct contact with the hearing nerve endings in the cochlea. Once placed in the inner ear and mastoid bone, these components are covered by the child's skin and hair. With the exception of the incision scar, and a small bump behind the ear, it will

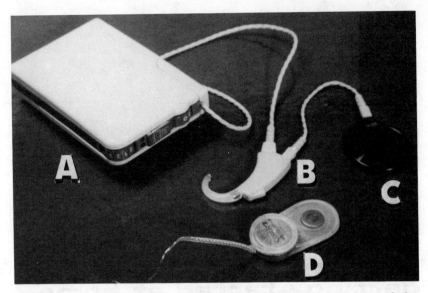

Figure 1–1:   The parts of the cochlear implant system are: a) the speech processor, b) the microphone, c) the transmitter coil, and d) the internal receiver and electrode array. A short cord connects the microphone to the transmitter coil. A longer cord connects the microphone to the speech processor.

not be obvious that the child has a cochlear implant when he is not wearing the external hardware.

Before the child can perceive sound with the implant, the internal components must be coupled with the externally worn parts of the implant system. The external components include a microphone, an external transmitter coil, cords, and a speech processor. They are fitted to the child approximately five weeks after surgery (Figure 1–1), when the incision site is well healed.

The implant microphone and external transmitter are worn on the child's head. The microphone looks like a behind-the-ear hearing aid and attaches over the child's pinna with an earhook. It receives the acoustic waveform and converts it into an electrical signal. It is connected by a short cord to the external transmitter which is about the size of a quarter.

A longer cord joins the microphone/transmitter to the speech processor. The speech processor is approximately the size of a cassette audio tape and can be worn any number of ways on the child's body. The processor contains the battery that powers the system, the user controls, and the software program that determines how incoming sound will be coded and transformed into electrical impulses.

Once incoming sound has been coded by the speech processor, the electrical signal travels back through the long cord to the external transmitter. The transmitter is a spoked ring with a magnet in the center. The attraction between this magnet and the internal magnet holds the transmitter against the child's head. The external transmitter communicates with the implanted part of the system through the child's hair and skin by means of high frequency radio waves. The radio signal is sent to the internal receiver where it is converted back into an electrical signal. The current travels to the electrodes and a unique pattern of stimulation occurs depending on the frequency and intensity characteristics of the incoming sound. From this point, the information about the sound travels through the auditory brainstem to the temporal lobe of the brain where sound is interpreted. Figure 1–2 shows how sound is transmitted through the implant system.

stimulating the implant

The process of fitting and adjusting the external components of the cochlear implant is often referred to as the tune-up. Most parents and children anxiously await the first tune-up session since it will be the child's first experience with sound through the implant. Because some children are unsure of what to expect, they may be frightened and reluctant to be fitted with the implant. Other children who are cognizant of their parents' excitement and expectations may find the process stressful. These feelings should be discussed when the parents and child are counseled and prepared by the audiologist for the first tune-up session. Table 1–1 presents some suggestions for parents to prepare themselves and their child for his first experience with sound through an implant.

The child and the audiologist must work closely together during the tune-up sessions. By means of a computer that interfaces with the implant system, the audiologist slowly increases the electrical current to each electrode until the child experiences some sensation of hearing (Figure 1–3). The child must indicate when sound is first perceived and when it is comfortably loud. Eventually all of the electrodes will be

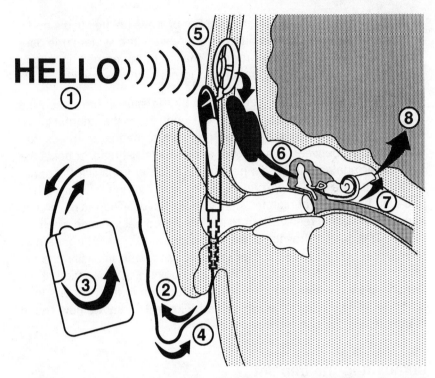

Figure 1–2: Sound transmission through the cochlear implant system: (1) Sound is received by the microphone and converted into an electrical signal. The signal travels via the long cord (2) to the speech processor which codes useful information (3). The coded signal travels back through the long cord (4) to the transmitter coil (5) which is magnetically attracted to the child's head. The signal passes through the child's skin by means of a high frequency radio signal to the internal receiver (6). Electrical signals are sent to the electrodes in the cochlea (7) where the hearing nerve endings are stimulated. This information travels to the auditory cortex where sound is interpreted.

stimulated and a range of soft to loud sound will be determined for each one. The audiologist then programs the speech processor using this information. This program can be modified and replaced as many times as needed. The audiologist must check and adjust the program several times during the first year as the child becomes accustomed to using the implant.

Table 1–1:   Suggestions for Preparing for the First Tune-Up.

The tune-up of the speech processor in a multichannel implant will require several visits to the implant center. Parents can prepare for the first tune-up session by following these recommendations:

A. Avoid a big build-up to the first tune-up session. Otherwise, the anticipation may be nerve-wracking for both parents and the child.

B. Leave siblings, grandparents and friends at home. It is usually better if just the parents are present.

C. Be prepared for the child to wear the speech processor by bringing a vest, harness or pocket T-shirt that will accommodate the device comfortably.

D. Bring the child's earmold that was used with his hearing aid for the implanted ear. The mold will help anchor the microphone and may make the child feel more secure about wearing the microphone/transmitter.

E. Bring along a few of the child's noisemaking toys. Once the speech processor is programmed, the child will be able to hear moderately soft sounds. A noisemaking toy is a good way to introduce the child to sound.

F. Counsel and prepare friends and family, especially grandparents, that the tune-up is only the first stage of the child's implant experience. The child must learn that sound is meaningful before he will respond to it; this will take months of time and practice.

For an implanted adult, the tuning of a multichannel implant takes about two to three hours. An older child who has a long attention span and understands what information the audiologist needs may require only slightly more time. For a young child, four to eight half-day sessions are usually required to tune the implant completely. Many deaf children find the concepts of soft and loud difficult to grasp. The child must learn what these concepts mean and apply them to the sensations he is experiencing. This requires considerable attention and concentration. Depending upon the age of the child, a number of techniques can be

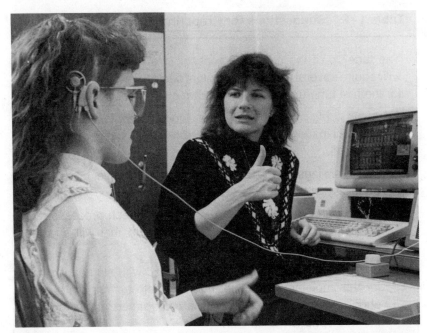

Figure 1–3a: An older child can tell the audiologist about the sound she is hearing when programming the speech processor.

used to help him learn how to reliably provide the necessary information. Toys and games are often used to help the child understand his task and make the tune-up process enjoyable.

Once the speech processor is programmed, the microphone/transmitter and the processor can be placed on the child. If the appropriate settings have been obtained, the child should be able to perceive moderately soft sounds, including speech, when the implant is turned on. Though he is able to *hear* sounds around him at this point, parents must recognize that they may not have meaning to the child, particularly if he was deafened early in life. Most newly implanted young children do not spontaneously react to sound until they learn to associate it with meaning. For example, a child will not recognize his name until he has heard it hundreds of times and learned to associate the sound pattern with its meaning. Children who had hearing prior to deafness will be more aware of sound and its meaning. In both cases the tune-up is just the beginning of the child's aural habilitation. A child's listening skills will unfold over the next months and years as he receives speech production and listening training and as his experience with sound increases.

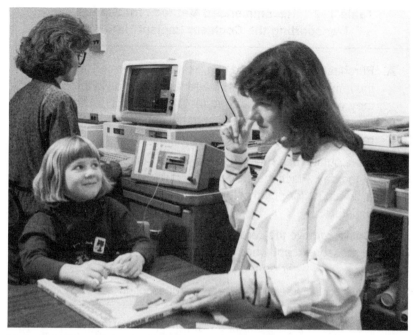

Figure 1–3b: Two clinicians are usually involved in programming the speech processor of a young child. One operates the computer which delivers the stimulation and the other interacts with the child.

caring for the implant

After the initial tune-up session, the child may begin wearing the implant components for moderated periods of time at home and at school. Table 1–2 includes recommended methods of storing and transporting the device.

The implant audiologist will demonstrate how to place the microphone/transmitter on the child's head and where to set the speech processor controls. Care of the implant will be discussed, including changing the batteries and troubleshooting techniques. The child and parents should practice putting on and removing the device, and changing the cords and batteries, several times under the audiologist's supervision. The parents, and eventually the child, must become comfortable handling and manipulating all the implant parts.

As with any well-used electronic device, malfunctions in the implant due to normal wear will occur. Parents must be proficient at diagnosing

**Table 1–2:   Recommended Methods for Storing and
Transporting the Cochlear Implant Hardware.**

A. Purchase a small padded bag, like a camera case, to transport
the implant parts. Put extra batteries and cords in the case so
they will be available if needed. This case should be used to
store the speech processor and microphone/transmitter when
removed from the child during the day.

B. Take out the batteries when the implant is removed at the end
of the day. Place the processor and microphone/transmitter in
a dri-aid kit for nightly storage to prevent breakdowns due to
moisture.

C. Do not remove the cords from the microphone and the speech
processor except when changing them. This will prevent unnecessary wear on the plugs and connectors.

D. If the child wears the speech processor in a pouch on his
chest, put it in a plastic bag before placing it in the pouch.
This will keep the processor dry from spills that invariably occur
when the child eats and drinks. A waterproof pocket flap will
also protect the processor.

---

problems so they can be remedied immediately. Appendix 1–1 includes
a checklist to assist them in finding and solving problems with the
implant equipment. The implant must be properly maintained so it can
be used on a regular basis.

While the manufacturer of the multichannel implant continually up-
grades parts to reduce the number of problems, it is inevitable that
breakdowns will occur, particularly with very active children.

wearing the implant

Once the implant has been programmed, the child should wear the
device every day. Putting on and using the cochlear implant will quickly
become routine, but the first few weeks the implant is worn may be a
time of great adjustment for the child. The parents must control or at
least supervise the placement and removal of the implant, depending

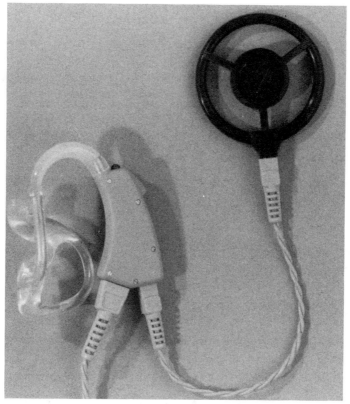

Figure 1–4: **A retainer mold, used to anchor the microphone to the child's ear.**

upon the age of the child. The first step in developing the new routine is to determine how the child will wear the external parts.

the microphone

The earhook holds the microphone over the child's pinna. Depending upon the child's activity, however, the earhook alone may not be adequate to keep the microphone in place. The audiologist may recommend that the child use an earmold to anchor the microphone. A retainer type of mold works well for this purpose since it secures the microphone and does not occlude the ear (Figure 1–4). The earmold tubing attaches to the microphone earhook as with a behind-the-ear hearing aid. Most audiologists can make or order this type of earmold.

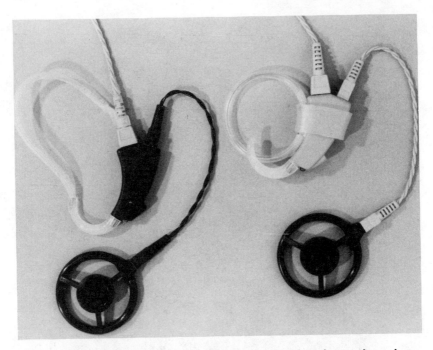

Figure 1–5: A Huggie and a Mic Lock, used to keep the microphone in place.

Another option for anchoring the microphone is use of a *Huggie*. It consists of a half-inch plastic band that holds the microphone and a pliable ring that encircles the child's pinna. Huggies of various sizes are available wherever hearing aid supplies are sold. Cochlear Corporation also makes a *Mic Lock* which is a piece of plastic tubing that attaches to the implant microphone and anchors it to the ear (Figure 1–5). The child may need to use a Huggie, Mic Lock or earmold only during rigorous activities.

the external transmitter

During the first few weeks of implant use the parents should check the site of the child's magnetic transmitter every day to ensure that the attraction between the internal and external magnet is secure and comfortable. If redness or tenderness develops around the site of the transmitter, the magnet may be too strong. Conversely, if the transmitter does not stay in place and falls off the child's head, the magnet may be too weak. In either case the cochlear implant audiologist should be contacted to change the magnet strength. Once the child's hair grows back around the incision site it may need to be trimmed occasionally to keep the transmitter securely in place. In most cases, use of the cochlear implant should not prevent a child from wearing his hairstyle as desired.

the cords

There are two important considerations regarding the cord that connects the microphone/transmitter to the processor. First, it must not impede the child's movement. Secondly, it must not get caught on the child or objects in his environment. There are several different lengths of cords available. The one that allows for freedom of movement without too much excess should be used. Placing the cord underneath clothing as it runs from the processor to the microphone/transmitter will prevent it from snagging on objects, which can damage the cord and processor.

the speech processor

Parents should select a secure yet comfortable way for the child to wear the speech processor. Depending upon the age of the child, he should help in this decision. In fact, the way the speech processor is worn should be considered even before the implant surgery so the child fully realizes how the implant will look. This is particularly important for adolescents who may be self-conscious about the appearance of the device. Children who have worn a body type hearing aid or a tactile device will find that the speech processor is about the same size and weight. It may be possible that the same pouch or harness used with these devices will hold the speech processor. The processor can be worn in a shirt or pants pocket if the pocket is fastened at the top and provides adequate support. A vest or harness worn close to the body will work best for young children. In some cases it may be necessary to place the speech processor out of the child's reach; for example, on a belt or in a harness on his back. This will prevent him from manipulating the controls and cords. Older children may prefer to wear the speech processor in a fanny pack around their waists. Whatever option is selected, the device should be comfortable to wear. Several possibilities may need to be explored before the final decision is made. Figures 1–6, (a-f). show alternatives for wearing the speech processor.

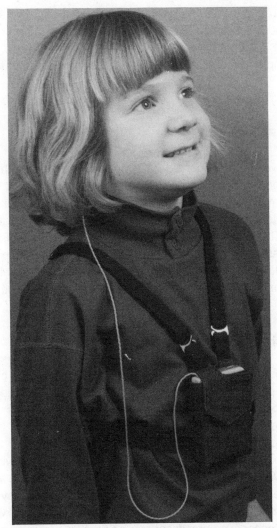

Figure 1–6a: Method of wearing the speech processor—in a chest harness.

The way the speech processor is worn may change with the child's activities. For some activities the speech processor must be more securely fitted and protected. For example, one teenage girl was the leading forward on her high school basketball team. She devised a special harness to wear under her uniform and used her implant during every game. For the senior prom, she and her mother created a special matching belt for her to wear the speech processor with her strapless gown.

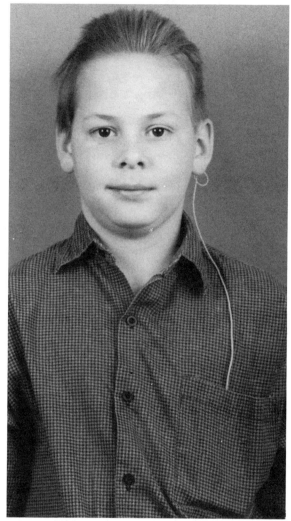

Figure 1–6b: **Method of wearing the speech processor—in a shirt pocket.**

special considerations

As the implanted child learns to depend on sound for communication, he will likely want to wear the device for all activities. However, because of the fragility of the external parts, precautions must be taken when wearing the device during rigorous physical activities. Use of a special harness and/or protective helmet may be necessary. In some cases

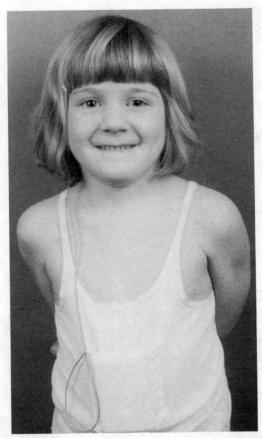

Figure 1–6c: Method of wearing the speech processor—in an undershirt pocket

the device will simply have to be removed. The processor and microphone/transmitter should be removed for bathing, swimming and sleeping. The child's physical limitations during the course of a school day should be discussed and parents should provide educators with guidelines (Chapter 2).

Many parents express concern for protecting the internal implant parts as well. Incidents of internal implant damage due to a direct blow to the side of the head have been reported but are rare. A helmet should be worn for any sporting activity that generally requires one, such as baseball, football or bicycling. A child's lifestyle should not be restricted because of the cochlear implant, but common sense must prevail. In

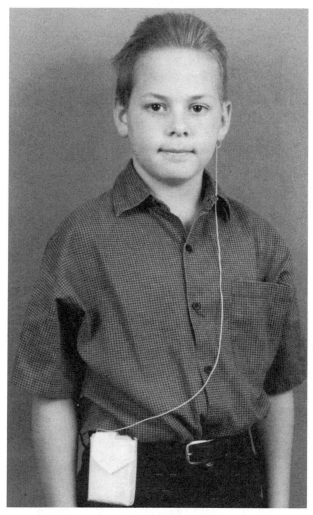

Figure 1–6d: Method of wearing the speech processor—in a belt pouch

the event of an accident, the internal implant components can be removed and replaced if necessary through a second operation.

There are several medical procedures that a person with a cochlear implant should not undergo. They include magnetic resonance imaging, electrosurgery, diathermy, electro-convulsive therapy, and ionizing radiation therapy. The implant surgeon will discuss these precautions with the family prior to surgery. The family pediatrician and dentist should be given

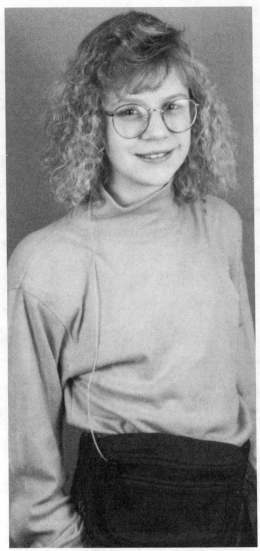

Figure 1–6e: Method of wearing the speech processor—in a fanny pack

copies of this information for the child's file. A patient identification card that includes this information is provided by the implant manufacturer and should be carried by the implant user. A Medic-Alert bracelet or pendant that identifies the wearer as an implant user is recommended for children. This jewelry can be ordered at most drugstores.

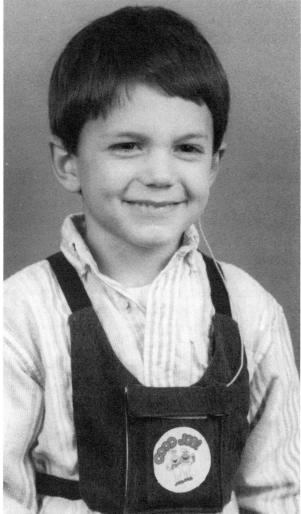

Figure 1–6f: Method of wearing the speech processor—in a vest-type pocket.

adjusting to sound

The time it takes for each child to adjust to the implant will vary. Parents must use their own judgement and knowledge of their child's behavior to make the transition into the world of sound a positive and pleasant experience. Most adult implant users require several weeks, if not months, to become comfortable wearing the implant. The child who has never heard before, or who has not heard for some time, may require more time. He may be overwhelmed by wearing a new apparatus and experiencing a new sensation. The adjustment period may be difficult not only for the child, but for the entire family since their routine and expectations of one another may change. To ease the transition, parents should provide guidelines for the child, establish a routine for wearing the implant, and optimize the child's listening and learning environment. They should also motivate the child to wear the device and support him with a positive attitude.

providing guidelines for implant use

Responsibility for handling the implant device will be shared by the parents, educators, and the child. The degree to which the young child is responsible, however, should be limited at first. The parents must provide guidelines for implant use. As a general rule, they should determine when the implant will be worn and when it will be removed. The parent or teacher should also initially be responsible for setting the speech processor controls. The recommended setting should be used at all times unless the environment includes a continuously loud noise. In those cases, the parent can temporarily turn off the processor or set it to a lower volume.

After the child has become accustomed to hearing, and wearing the implant is routine, he can be given more independence. In the meantime, the parent should ensure that the child does not alter the device settings. For example, one implanted child was not showing any sign of sound awareness after six months of implant use. For months his parents and teachers alerted him to sound and he smiled and nodded as if he had heard it. When he continually failed to independently acknowledge the presence of sound, they observed him more closely and discovered he was turning the processor off or down. He had to be taught that adjusting the processor settings was not allowed unless he first asked his parent or teacher. Within a short period of time, with regular exposure to sound, he began to respond to sounds without prompting and could truly share his parents' and teacher's enthusiasm for hearing.

Older children may be given more autonomy with the implant, but should be encouraged to wear it as much as possible at the recommended settings. The child should understand that he is expected to wear the implant regularly and that the more he wears it, the greater the benefits will ultimately be. Ideally, the child will want to wear the implant; realistically, it may be a point of contention for the family and will therefore require some persistent encouragement and reinforcement.

establish a routine for wearing the device

For the first few weeks, the parents and child should establish a minimum amount of time the implant will be worn each day. This will vary from day to day as the time gradually increases. Initially, a realistic goal is twenty or thirty minutes, several times a day. As the child becomes accustomed to hearing, he will tolerate longer periods of stimulation. Wearing the implant for long periods of time before he has developed a tolerance may result in unpleasant reactions. Some adult users have commented that the implant causes tinnitus or ringing in their ears and head when first used. Others have found that use of the implant makes them irritable or easily fatigued. Some report headaches. These problems are usually overcome with experience. For the first several weeks, parents should observe their child for signs of unusual behavior, including aggressiveness and irritability, and alter the use of the implant as needed.

Eventually, the child should wear the implant during all waking hours. Consistent use is essential to maximize the benefits of implantation. Audition will become an integral part of the child's communication ability only if his listening skills are nurtured and developed. In general, full-time use of the implant should be achieved within two months after the initial stimulation.

optimize the listening environment

Because sound may initially overwhelm the new implant user, he should begin wearing the device in relatively quiet settings. The variety of settings will expand naturally as the length of time the child uses the implant increases. Parents should not require the child to wear the implant in noisy environments such as a shopping center or church for the first few weeks. The presence of sound from unknown sources may be frightening or confusing. The goal is to make hearing a pleasant experience. Chapter 4 presents strategies for structuring the environment to promote successful listening and speechreading.

motivate the child to learn

The best way to motivate a child to use the implant is to make listening fun and rewarding. As he learns to identify meaningful sounds, the child will be encouraged by his abilities, particularly when his parents react positively. When increasing his use time or providing auditory training, parents should keep the child's interests in mind. They should find board games that the child enjoys, and include activities and conversational topics that interest him. Even if the child will use the implant for only a short period of time he should be praised for his achievement. Once the child becomes accustomed to hearing and uses the implant routinely, the need for direct reinforcement will subside. Siblings or playmates may be included in activities to make learning more fun. This will also teach them how to communicate effectively with the implanted child.

maintain a positive attitude

Parents should demonstrate an enthusiastic and optimistic attitude about the child's use of the cochlear implant. Children are perceptive to their parents' feelings. If the parent views training with the implant as a chore or treats the implant hardware as a burden to bear, the child will react similarly. The development of auditory skills is a slow process and cannot be accomplished by the child independently. He will need support, guidance, and much supervised practice to learn to use sound meaningfully. The child will encounter growth spurts and plateaus in his auditory development. Maintaining a positive yet realistic attitude will help parents weather those periods when the child seems to make little or no progress.

All parents want their child to have a positive self image. The self image reflects the child's feelings of acceptance and worth. When parents project a positive attitude about the child's use of the implant, he learns to accept the implant as part of himself. One parent of an implanted child proudly reported about an open house she attended at her son's school. Each child in his class drew a self portrait to hang outside the classroom for the occasion. Her son included in great detail the speech processor and microphone/transmitter in his portrait. This self-portrait demonstrated the child's positive image of himself and the acceptance of his cochlear implant (Figure 1–7).

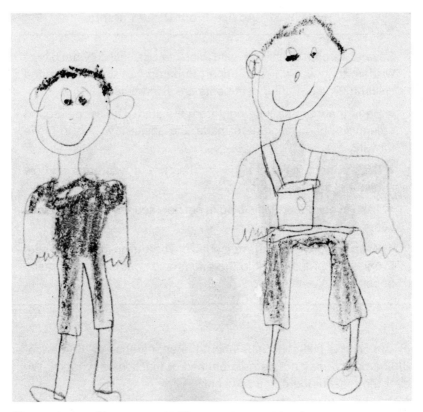

Figure 1-7: **Five-year-old Tim produced this picture when asked to draw himself with his best friend.**

Table 1-3 presents advice that parents of implant users would offer to other parents.

resistance to using the implant

No matter how enthusiastic and supportive the parents are, some children will resist wearing and using the implant. In these cases, it is particularly important for parents to make rules and provide reinforcement.

Parents should identify the reason for the child's noncompliance. Most reasons for resisting the implant arise from one of the following situations: a) the child feels uncomfortable with the physical arrangement of the device, b) the child is unaccustomed to the presence of sound,

Table 1–3:   Advice From Other Parents.

Several parents of children with implants were asked what bits of wisdom they would like to impart to parents of newly implanted children. Some of their comments are listed below:

●"Be firm about use time right from the start. The sooner sound recognition connections are made, the easier it will be to move forward."

●"Don't expect major changes at the start. It was amazing how subtle the changes were."

●"Take every opportunity to point out new sounds and where they come from."

●"Keep your expectations reasonable. There is no magic involved. Progress is proportional to the efforts and contributions of many people."

c) the child is self-conscious about the appearance of the device, or d) the device may not be programmed or functioning properly. Whatever the reason, there is a solution.

In cases where the child is not comfortable wearing the hardware, the parents should experiment with various ways of wearing the device. For instance, they might purchase a special belt or make a lightweight harness. One parent made inexpensive colored pouches that matched several of her daughter's outfits.

When the child reacts adversely to the presence of sound, the parents should ease the child into the routine of wearing the implant by limiting the use time and then expanding it gradually. For a young child, the parents may mark time with a cooking timer and make a reinforcement book with stickers and privileges to be won when the designated time is over. It may be necessary for the child to wear the device, but have it turned off or set at a lower volume until he is used to the physical arrangement of wearing the implant and the presence of sound. However, the recommended setting should be used as soon as possible.

When the child is self-conscious about the implant, the parents and child should discuss the child's feelings. Parents should explain why the implant is important and how it will help the child. The parent might plan a special excursion that includes having the child wear the device. The parents should show pride in the child's use of the implant and expect him to wear it regularly. With the appropriate attention and re-inforcement, an understanding can be achieved.

Finally, if the child continues to resist the device the audiologist should be consulted to determine if the speech processor program is appropriate. Sound may be too loud for the child or a part of the device may be malfunctioning and in need of repair.

enhancing speechreading

supplement sign language

Part of the process of selecting appropriate candidates for cochlear implantation includes determining whether or not conventional ampli-fication is helpful to a child. Children who ultimately receive implants are those who are unable to use hearing aids to detect and understand speech or environmental sounds. Because these children have heard very little prior to receiving the implant, they may be unprepared or unable to attend to sound. They may not realize that sound is meaningful when the implant is introduced, particularly if they were born deaf or lost their hearing at an early age. These children have likely been using sign language to communicate. Because this is the foundation of their ability to express themselves and to receive information, it would be inappropriate to stop signing once they receive an implant (Chapter 4). Sound must be integrated into their communication mode. Most children who receive cochlear implants will continue to be highly dependant upon sign language. The implant may afford increased independence, however, by allowing the children to hear speech and other sounds, and speechread others more successfully.

incorporate speechreading and audition into communication

The primary benefit of cochlear implantation for adults is speechreading enhancement (Chapter 7). The electrical signal from the implant alone is too incomplete to allow most adult users to understand speech in an audition only condition. However, when the electrical signal is paired with lipreading, most adult implant users can participate in normal con-versations. To realize similar kinds of benefits, the child's speech perception training should focus on the development of his speechreading skills along with his listening skills. To nurture these undeveloped abilities in the new implant user, practice in speechreading and listening, without sign, should be accomplished on a regular basis. Practice may take place as the child and his parents complete their daily routines and activities. Alternatively, practice may be accomplished with planned exercises or games. Depending upon the age of the child, all practice activities should be planned with the child's interests and abilities in mind. Chapters 5, 6, and 7 include discussion of informal and formal auditory and speechreading training techniques.

summary

When parents choose to pursue cochlear implantation for their deaf child, they embark on a decision that will impact the rest of their lives. Understanding how the implant works and optimizing the child's use of the device is the parents' responsibility. They must help the child accept the device and learn to use sound meaningfully. Ensuring that the implant components are comfortably fitted and are well maintained will ease the child's transition into the world of sound. Providing opportunities for listening practice and reinforcing the child's use of the implant will nurture his developing auditory skills. As the child learns to listen, the implant will become an integral part of his ability to communicate.

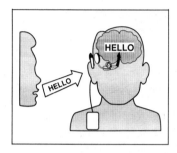

2

the implanted child at school

holly fryauf-bertschy, m.a.
karen iler kirk, ph.d.

The needs of a child with an implant are similar to those of a moderately to severely hearing-impaired child who uses hearing aids. The classroom teacher has a vital role in helping the child learn to adjust to the implant and use sound. This can be a learning process for the teacher as well as the student. This chapter discusses the implant hardware and how to maintain it. Suggestions for orienting the child to sound and evaluating his abilities are included. The role of the speech-language pathologist is also considered.

educational goals

There are two general educational goals for a deaf child. The first is for the child to develop his language and communication skills to the greatest extent possible. The second is for the child to master the same academic materials as his normal hearing peers (Moore, 1985). Technological advances in assistive devices, including hearing aids, tactile devices, and cochlear implants, should facilitate achieving these goals. These devices allow teachers, speech-language pathologists, and aural rehabilitationists to implement more effectively academic and habilitative programs. Minimally, the cochlear implant provides sound detection for the child who cannot otherwise perceive sound. With more information available to the child, formal instruction is facilitated. Incidental or spontaneous learning through hearing may also occur when the child learns to attend to and interpret the electrical signal.

implant systems for children

Several types of cochlear implants are available for adults, but only two systems are used by children in the United States. The 3M/House single-channel cochlear implant was the first to be approved by the United States Food and Drug Administration for use by children. However, it is no longer available for new patients. Presently, the Cochlear Corporation Nucleus implant is the most commonly implanted device. It was approved by the Food and Drug Administration on June 28, 1990 for general use by deaf children between two and seventeen years of age. The Nucleus device utilizes twenty-two electrodes that are placed in the cochlea. The speech processor codes the overall amplitude of the signal, fundamental frequency (voice pitch), and spectral peaks that correspond to the first two vowel formants (Chapter 6). There are two versions of the Nucleus multichannel implant: the Wearable Speech Processor (WSP) and the Mini Speech Processor (MSP). The WSP was updated and replaced by the MSP in early 1990. In addition to the information coded by the WSP, the MSP codes three bands of high frequency energy, which may allow the user to perceive acoustic information associated with some consonants, and the third vowel formant.

accepting the cochlear implant in the classroom

When a student receives a cochlear implant, the classroom teacher has the unique opportunity to watch the child's auditory skills develop and unfold on a daily basis. She can observe the child who was previously oblivious to sound, learn to incorporate sound into his everyday routines. Most teachers find this an exciting and interesting process. Handling the implant device and helping the child learn to adjust to his new sense may be intimidating to some teachers at first. The teacher can obtain technical support regarding the implant from the cochlear implant center. Many centers will provide videotaped and printed materials and/or an inservice to the school. Information from the center will assist the teacher in becoming comfortable with the child's use of the implant in the classroom.

checking and handling the implant hardware

Although the cochlear implant system is the result of sophisticated technology, using the device is very simple. Several teachers report that checking and maintaining the implant hardware is less difficult than maintaining the classroom FM system. Just as she ensures the hearing aids and auditory trainers of her students are in good working order, the teacher should also become familiar with the basic functioning of the implant and become proficient at identifying when a problem exists.

While it is not necessary for the teacher to know the technical aspects of the implant sound coding strategies, she should understand how sound is processed through the implant system (Figure 1–2, p.4). Sound waves are picked up by the ear-level microphone and converted to electrical current. Instead of being amplified and passed through the outer and middle ear, as with a hearing aid, the electrical signal is transmitted by a cord to the speech processor. The speech processor works like a small computer. It analyzes the incoming signal and codes the fundamental frequency and the bands of acoustic energy or formant frequencies of the sound or voice. Gross characteristics about the duration and loudness of the signal are coded too. The coded signal is then sent to the transmitter coil by cords. The transmitter coil converts the electrical signal to a high frequency radio signal that passes through the child's skin to the implanted receiver. The receiver decodes the signal and sends electrical impulses to the appropriate electrodes. Each electrode is tuned to a narrow band of frequencies. The electrodes directly stimulate the auditory nerve endings. This stimulation pattern is carried through the auditory nervous system to the auditory cortex where sound is interpreted. The coding and transmission of sound through the implant system happens instantaneously.

the function check

Hearing aids or auditory trainers can be listened to with a hearing aid stethoscope to ensure that they are functioning properly. Unfortunately,

**Table 2–1:   The Daily Function Check for the Cochlear
Corporation Nucleus Cochlear Implant
(the MSP or WSP Speech Processor).**

A. Set the speech processor to "T" for test. The red light at the
top of the processor should shine continuously.

B. With an MSP, place the child's transmitter coil against the front
center, near the top, of the speech processor. With processor
on user settings, the "C" for coil light should flicker continuously. With a WSP, place the check wand against the coil and
watch for the red light in the center to flicker.

C. Set the processor to user settings. Hold the microphone approximately one foot from your mouth and say the Ling Five-
Sounds. In a quiet setting, the "M" for microphone light should
flicker for each sound.

---

a "listening check" cannot be performed with a cochlear implant. Only
the implanted child can hear through the system. Each implant user
has unique perceptual abilities that are determined by his residual hearing, his previous experience with sound, and his ability to use the electrical signal.

While it is not possible to know exactly what the child is perceiving, the
teacher can ensure that the implant is functioning appropriately by completing a simple daily function check of the implant (Table 2–1). This
simple check, which is similar to a hearing aid check, requires only a
few minutes to complete. It should be part of the daily classroom routine.
The implant function check is particularly important for young children,
who may not reliably report a malfunction. Older children may complete
the check themselves, with the teacher's supervision.

If the function check indicates the implant is not working correctly, the
teacher can identify the source of the problem by methodically checking
each part following the Classroom Troubleshooting Guide (Table 2–2).
The first step is to ensure that cords are plugged in correctly and securely and that the appropriate device settings are used. If the problem
still exists, the teacher can try two repairs. First, she can check the
battery to see if it is properly charged, and replace it if necessary. After

Table 2–2: Classroom Troubleshooting Guide for the Cochlear Corporation Nucleus Device (The MSP or WSP Processor).

A. Check each component to ensure it is correctly and securely coupled to the adjacent part. The polarity of the long cord is indicated by a dot on the connector plug. Match it to the dot on the microphone. The right angled connector which plugs into the speech processor can fit in only one way on the MSP. On the WSP, match the dot on the plug to the dot on the adaptor to the speech processor.

B. Set the processor control to "T" for test. The red "M" light on the top of the processor should shine continuously. If the child is wearing the device, he should hear a steady sound. Confirm this. If the light does not come on or the child does not hear the sound, change the battery.

C. With the MSP, place the child's transmitter coil against the front center, near the top, of the speech processor. Turn the implant controls to the user setting. The "C" light on the speech processor should flicker continuously. With the WSP, place the check wand against the coil and watch for the red light to flicker. If the "C" light or the wand light does not flicker, change the long cord and recheck. Next, change the short cord from the transmitter coil to the microphone and recheck.

D. If after completing all the steps above, the device is nonfunctional or the child reports he cannot hear or that the sound quality is poor, contact his parents so they can call the implant center.

---

replacing a bad battery, she should repeat the function check. The second possible repair is to change the cords. The long cord that couples the microphone to the speech processor should be replaced first. If the device is still nonfunctional, the short cord that connects the microphone and transmitter coil can be replaced. A spare set of cords and batteries provided by the child's parents should be kept at school so they will be available when needed. If problems still exist after troubleshooting, the teacher should contact the child's parents so they can call the implant center immediately. When spare batteries and cords are used at school, the teacher can notify the parents for replacements.

using the implant at school

Just as she monitors the other students' use of hearing aids, the teacher must ensure that the child is using the cochlear implant properly. The microphone/transmitter and speech processor should be placed and set appropriately. The microphone, which looks like a behind-the-ear hearing aid, is placed over the child's pinna and may be anchored by an earmold. The transmitter coil, which is connected to the microphone by a short cord, attaches by magnetic attraction to the components implanted in the child's mastoid area behind the ear. The coil will stay in position only when placed in the proper location. The attraction between the internal and external magnet will make this location obvious. The child's parents are responsibile for providing the child with a safe and comfortable means of wearing the speech processor. They should also provide the teacher with information regarding the appropriate settings of the speech processor and a strategy for building the child's use time.

When a child first receives an implant, he must adjust to the physical arrangement of the device and to the presence of sound. Parents are instructed by the implant audiologist to increase gradually the time the child wears the implant each day during the first month of use. Initially, the teacher should expect the young child to wear the implant turned on for several short periods of time during the school day, typically thirty to forty-five minutes. The child must develop a tolerance to electrical stimulation. If he exhibits signs of unusual fatigue or irritability, his use time should be reduced and then increased gradually. Within approximately two months of the initial stimulation, full-time use should be expected.

The child should wear the implant only for selected activities initially; for example, during speech therapy or story time, and during small group or individual activities. Background noise should be minimized as much as possible. The child should have access to visual speech cues, contextual cues, and sign (if appropriate), to supplement the sound he is hearing. After the adjustment period, when the child is more comfortable wearing the implant, he will learn to attend to meaningful sounds and tune out much of the normal classroom noise.

The teacher and speech-language pathologist should remember that the child may not spontaneously react to sound initially, particularly if he has been deaf for some time. Consistent auditory stimulation should be provided to the child, but expectations for his response to sound should be minimal. Once the child has become accustomed to hearing and the teacher and speech-language pathologist have had the chance to evaluate his skills, realistic speech perception and production objectives can be developed.

exceptions to regular use

If the implant hardware is at risk of falling off or being damaged in physical activities, as in gym class or during recess, it should be removed. An older child will learn to identify situations when the implant hardware should not be worn. Parents should be consulted to establish guidelines for removing the device of a younger child. When the implant is removed during the school day, it should be placed in the child's carrying case (Chapter 1) and stored in a safe place. While it is important to protect the implant hardware from unnecessary wear and tear, no learning of environmental sounds or aural/oral exchange with other children can occur if the child is not wearing the device.

The external hardware is not waterproof. If the child goes outside in the rain, the device should be protected with a raincoat and hat, or removed. The teacher may need to monitor the young child's use of the drinking fountain and restroom. He can wear the implant during lunch time if it is protected from spills. If the child wears the speech processor on his chest, it can be protected from food and drink by placing it in a plastic sandwich bag within the harness. A vest with a waterproof pocket flap will protect the processor as well.

Many teachers express concern for the safety of the internal or implanted components of the system. The internal receiver/stimulator is susceptible to damage if the child sustains a direct blow to the side of the head. If he engages in activities that include use of a hard ball, such as baseball or football, the child should wear a protective helmet. The implanted child should be discouraged from wrestling or rough play. School personnel who are responsibile for the child during recess and gym class should be informed of the child's restrictions regarding physical activities.

familiarizing classmates with the implant

The implanted child's classmates will be curious about his special device. Initially, the implant will be the source of many questions. Intro-

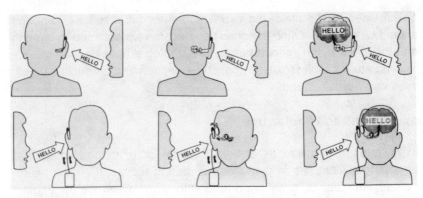

Figure 2–1: This illustration compares a hearing aid to a cochlear implant. In both cases, the microphone picks up sound. With a hearing aid (top), amplified sound travels through the middle ear to the cochlea. With a cochlear implant (bottom), sound is coded by the speech processor. The signal is then transmitted through the child's head to the implanted electrodes in the cochlea.

ducing the implant and describing it as another type of hearing aid will help other students understand its function. The teacher can use the illustrations in Figure 2–1 to explain how the cochlear implant compares to a conventional behind-the-ear hearing aid. An older child may be encouraged to provide a short presentation about the implant. A younger child can present the implant for "show and tell". The implant will eventually become an accepted and unremarkable part of the classroom environment.

using the implant with FM systems

An FM system can be coupled to the cochlear implant system to compensate for distance, noise, and reverberation problems within the classroom. The FM unit transmits the signal from the teacher's microphone, or a sound source, by radio frequency to the child's receiver. The child's receiver or auditory trainer receives and amplifies the signal. When used with a cochlear implant, little amplification is necessary since the speech processor codes the relative intensity of incoming sounds. A special cord must be obtained from the implant center or the FM unit manufacturer to successfully couple the two systems. Figure 2–2 indicates how sound is transmitted from the source to the child's

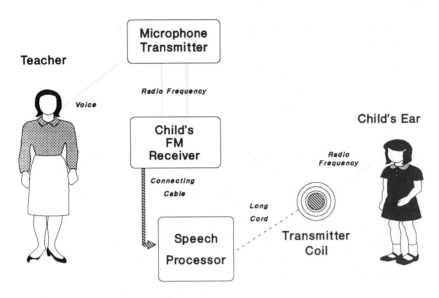

Figure 2–2: The transmission of sound from the teacher, through the FM system, to the child using a cochlear implant.

implant. A step-by-step process for adjusting the FM unit and coupling it to the speech processor is included in Appendix 2–1.

Before deciding to use the FM system with an implant, the teacher must consider three factors. The first factor is whether or not the classroom activities and environment necessitate the use of an FM system. In small or self-contained classrooms, the teacher may work closely with her students. She may engage in small group and one-to-one activities and present few formal lectures. There may be no significant distance problems to overcome. Many self-contained classrooms are treated to control for noise and reverberation. Use of an FM system may not significantly improve the child's listening environment beyond using the implant alone. The time and trouble of maintaining the FM unit may not be justified.

The second factor to consider is whether or not the child can indicate when he is experiencing a hardware problem. When the FM system is coupled to the implant, the potential for hardware problems increases two-fold. The FM system may introduce sound distortion from over-amplification or interference from other radio signals. Until the child can reliably report a problem with his implant, the FM system should not be coupled to it. The child should be able to indicate whether the sound quality with the FM system is comparable to using the implant alone.

The final factor to consider before using an FM system is whether or not the child will tolerate it. There must be room for him to comfortably wear both the implant hardware and the FM receiver.

combining communication and academic goals

The school day for the hearing impaired child is full. Conceivably, the entire day could be spent on communication-centered activities such as language development, auditory and speechreading training, speech production, and communication therapy. It is an ongoing challenge for the teacher of the hearing-impaired to set and achieve goals in these areas as well as complete the necessary academic studies. The teacher must combine communication exercises and academic coursework whenever possible.

Auditory training and speechreading training can be incorporated into academic studies. When developing lesson plans, the teacher should consider how the child might practice listening and speechreading during the lesson. For example, a U.S. geography lesson involving locating states on the map can include a speechreading activity. The teacher can ask the child to speechread her as she says the name of a state. He must then spell the name and locate the state on the map. For another example, the teacher might incorporate auditory training into a language lesson concerning verb endings. The child must read a base sentence from the chalkboard. The teacher then restates the sentence in a different form; for example, *The boy sits*, versus *The boy is sitting*, versus *The boy sat*. The child listens and is asked to identify which form of the verb was used.

Vocabulary and materials from academic lessons can make auditory and speechreading training exercises meaningful and relevant. For example, the teacher may use vocabulary from the current social studies lesson on American Indians for an auditory training task. The child can discriminate the name of tools used by the Indians. The teacher can use spelling words during a speechreading exercise. She can ask the student to speechread the word and then spell it correctly. Vocabulary words from completed language lessons can be reviewed when used for speechreading and auditory training exercises.

evaluating the child's abilities with the cochlear implant

Formal and informal testing will help the teacher understand the student's unique auditory abilities. The results of testing will provide the teacher with information that will affect her interactions with and expectations of the child in all classroom activities. Evaluation is an ongoing process as the child's communication skills develop.

informal assessment techniques

The teacher should continually assess a child's abilities with informal tests and observations. Detection tasks will indicate the child's ability to perceive sounds of different intensity or loudness, pitch, and temporal pattern. Most cochlear implant users can detect the presence of speech when it is as soft as 40 to 50 dB HL, which is the level of quiet, conversational speech.

In the classroom the child's detection range can be tested. Once the child can reliably respond to a stimulus, such as his name, he can sit at his desk, listen for the teacher to say his name, and raise his hand when he hears it. The teacher then moves around the room, says the child's name, and notes his responses. Initially, the child may detect the teacher's voice, but may not recognize his own name. With time and practice, the child may learn to respond to his name within that range, if he is not too engrossed in an activity and if background noise is minimal.

Another informal test of speech sound perception is the *Ling Five-Sounds-Test* (Ling, 1988). The child claps his hands when he hears the teacher produce /u/ (boot), /a/ (pop), /i/ (beat), /ʃ/ (shhh), and /s/ (sss). Detection of these five sounds implies that the child perceives information across the speech frequencies, 250 Hz to 6,000 Hz. If detection is possible, the teacher can next evaluate the child's ability to discriminate and then identify the sounds.

The teacher should continually observe the child's responses to environmental sounds. She should note the child's ability to detect sound when background noise is present. Noise competes with other incoming signals and decreases the child's abilities to perceive speech and environmental sounds. For example, a child who typically responds to his name in quiet may have great difficulty detecting and discriminating it when classmates are active and noisy. Whenever possible, the child

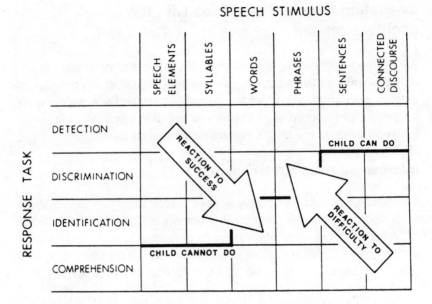

Figure 2–3:   The Erber model of auditory training.

should be positioned so that visual cues are maximized and competing noise is minimized.

As the child's auditory skills develop, the implanted child will begin to depend on sound for communication. Some of the secondary benefits of audition, such as improved speech and language, often appear after the child has used the implant for several months. By observing the child interact with other children, both hearing and hearing-impaired, the teacher will appreciate how well the child is hearing and communicating.

formal assessment techniques

Several tests and therapy tools are available for screening the child's discrimination, identification and comprehension skills. Appendix 2–2 lists some commercially available tools for assessing and developing auditory skills. The results of these tests can guide the teacher in designing auditory training and speechreading training objectives.

The Erber Model of Auditory Training (Erber, 1982) (Figure 2–3) is an assessment technique that can be used to develop appropriate speechreading and auditory training lessons. The objective in using this adaptive model is to determine what perceptual tasks the child can easily accomplish and what he cannot accomplish. Subsequent training should then focus along that boundary. The teacher adaptively chooses training materials based on the child's success or difficulty with the previous stimuli. For example, if a child can speechread single words, but not sentence-length materials, short phrases can be used during speech-reading training. Phrases will be challenging, but will allow the child to experience some success. Response tasks can be determined adaptively as well. If the child can discriminate whether two short phrases are the same or different, the teacher should attempt an identification task where the child selects the appropriate picture after hearing the phrase.

the role of the speech-language pathologist

The speech-language pathologist is an important resource for the child with a cochlear implant. She supplements the work of the teacher with intensive and personalized communication activities for the child. The hearing-impaired child presents a unique and difficult challenge to most school speech-language pathologists. Not only do most children have major language deficits, but their speech production skills are also poor. The speech-language pathologist must assess the implanted child's speech and language abilities and provide appropriate remediation. Additionally, she assists teachers and parents in setting suitable goals and incorporating speech and/or language instruction into the child's daily activities. To fulfill these roles, the speech-language pathologist must understand what information is normally available in the speech signal, how a hearing loss can affect the use of this information, and which speech cues are available through the implant.

assessing speech and language skills

An assessment of the implanted child's speech and language skills should include both formal and informal measures. Any evaluation should be conducted in the child's primary communication mode. An interpreter should be employed as necessary to ensure that the implanted child understands the tasks, and that the results reflect the child's true abilities.

Formal assessment procedures are useful in determining the child's present skills and in identifying remediation goals. Appendix 2–3 provides a list of speech and language tests that are sometimes used with implanted children. Whenever possible, tests that have been specifically developed for hearing-impaired students should be employed. Test measures with normative data for normal-hearing children can also be useful in determining how the child's performance compares with his normal-hearing peers. However, caution must be used in interpreting the results of such tests because the manner of test presentation may differ from that used during test standardization. For example, signed instructions might accompany oral instructions. Furthermore, it is inappropriate to assign any sort of "mental age" to the implanted child that is based upon data from normal-hearing children. Instead, test results should be used to identify age-appropriate skills acquired by the implanted child, and those in need of remediation.

During formal assessment children are most likely to use the speech and language skills they have acquired. Until such skills are firmly established they may not generalize to less structured situations. Analyzing a sample of the child's spontaneous productions helps determine whether skills exhibited during testing appear in a less formal setting. In addition, the speech-language pathologist should observe the child interacting with his teacher, peers, and parents if possible. Such observations will enable her to develop strategies for promoting generalization of speech and language skills.

remediating speech skills

A discussion of speech remediation is beyond the scope of this chapter. However, we suggest that in establishing a remediation plan for the implanted child the speech-language pathologist should keep in mind the speech contrasts preserved by the implant processor. Chapters 6 and 7 describe the acoustic information available through the implant and relate this to the perception of different speech sound classes.

Speaking and listening are not isolated events. In many ways, the early stages of speech training and auditory training are parallel. For example, initial auditory training tasks may require the child to make gross sound discriminations among the prosodic speech aspects such as *long* versus *short*, *loud* versus *soft*, and *high* versus *low*. Likewise, an initial goal of speech instruction is mastery of these contrasts in a speech context. Other early auditory training exercises include awareness, discrimination, and identification of vowels. Similarly, vowel production initially preceeds consonant production in speech instruction. Incorporating listening practice into speech therapy, and speaking exercises into auditory training, increases practice opportunities and develops the child's ability to monitor his own speech.

interacting with parents and teachers

Speech and language skills will develop and generalize to many communication settings if the child has numerous opportunities for practicing them throughout the day. Teachers and parents must constantly provide good speech models, whether or not they are accompanied by signs. They must also encourage the child to verbalize for all communication.

The speech-language pathologist can facilitate the transfer of these skills by serving as a resource person to parents and teachers. She should familiarize them with the natural progression of speech and language skills, and with the child's current abilities. When the initial assessment has been completed, the speech-language pathologist should inform parents and teachers of her therapy goals for the child. After each therapy session, notes should be made describing the child's progress. These can be kept in a notebook and regularly shared with parents and teachers.

As the child acquires new skills, suggestions for promoting speech production outside of the therapy setting should be provided to parents and teachers. For example, as new speech sounds are acquired the speech-language pathologist can send home lists of practice items with these sounds. Practice materials should increase in complexity as the child's skills increase. Thus the child may practice syllables, words, phrases, and then sentences with the intended sounds. The child can practice exercise lists by playing games such as *Sound Bingo* or *Sound Tic-Tac-Toe*. The intended target (sound, word, or phrase) must be correctly produced before a marker is placed on the game board. Such activities give the child a chance to use his new skills with siblings, friends, and classmates, which promotes generalization. For sentence-level practice the speech-language pathologist can provide parents simple stories containing many examples of the target sounds. Parents can also help the child write his own story. Initially the opportunity to practice new skills in this way can be fun and reinforcing for the child. However, the production of new skills cannot be limited to formal activities. As the production of new skills becomes firmly established, one should expect some spontaneous transfer to natural communication (Ling, 1976). Parents and teachers should encourage the child to use his new skills, particularly during routine daily activities.

The speech-language pathologist should be an active participant in the implanted child's habilitation. She and the teacher can work together to implement an integrated remediation plan incorporating both speech and auditory training activities. Additionally, by educating parents about speech and language development, and by providing them with suggestions or materials for home use, the generalization of newly acquired speech and language skills will be maximized.

summary

The classroom teacher and speech-language pathologist can have a great impact on a child's successful use of a cochlear implant. As the number of children receiving implants increases, teachers will become experienced in working with these children and their special hardware. This chapter provides information about handling and maintaining the implant and helping the child learn to adjust to hearing.

references

Berg, F.S. (1987). *Facilitating Classroom Listening*. Boston: College Hill Press.

Erber, M.P. (1982). *Auditory Training*. Washington, D.C.: Alexander Graham Bell Association for the Deaf, Inc.

Ling, D. (1976). *Speech and the Hearing-Impaired Child: Theory and Practice*. Washington, D.C: Alexander Graham Bell Association for the Deaf, Inc.

Ling, D. (1988). *Foundations of Spoken Language for Hearing Impaired Children*. Washington, D.C.: Alexander Graham Bell Association for the Deaf, Inc.

Moores, D.F. (1985). Educational programs and services for hearing impaired children: issues and options. In F. Powell, T. Finitzo-Hieber, S. Friel-Patti, D. Henderson (Eds.) *Education of the Hearing Impaired Child*, (pp 3–20), San Diego: College-Hill Press.

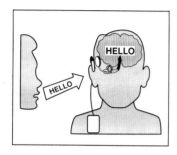

3

hearing abilities of children with cochlear implants

richard s. tyler, ph.d.
holly fryauf-bertschy, m.a.

The cochlear implant is designed to improve hearing. While we hope that there will be improvements in the child's speech production skills, language, cognition, and socialization, these will be secondary benefits from the hearing provided by the cochlear implant (Figure 3–1).

There are several important reasons to evaluate the perceptual abilities of children with cochlear implants. Perceptual evaluation is necessary to document the progress of the child, to ensure that the device is functioning appropriately, and to plan aural rehabilitation. It is also necessary for determining who is and who is not an appropriate cochlear implant candidate at the pre-implant stage. Because cochlear implants are new instruments (compared to hearing aids), they have been used by children for a relatively short period of time. There is much to learn about the effects of implantation on a recipient's educational, social, and communicative development. As with adult implant users, children vary greatly in their performance. Understanding the variables that influence performance may

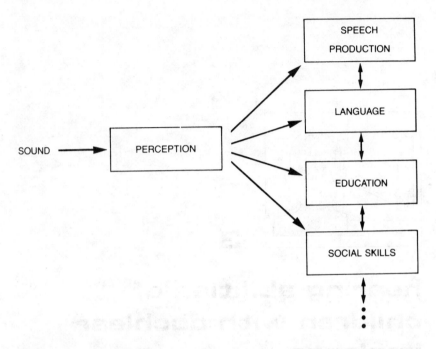

Figure 3–1: **A schematic display of the potential areas where cochlear implants could benefit a child. Because the cochlear implant allows the child to perceive sound, expect to observe initial improvement in hearing skills. Other improvements, such as in speech production, should follow, although these other areas are influenced by many other factors. From Tyler et. al. (1985) with permission.**

help us appreciate why some children use implants successfully, while others achieve less success overall.

audiological data

the audiogram

One of the basic measures of hearing ability is the audiogram (Figure 3–2). The audiogram is a graph that reflects the child's ability to detect sounds at different frequencies. The lowest level at which the child can detect a sound is recorded for each ear. This hearing test is usually performed either under earphones (unaided), or without earphones in a sound treated room (in the sound field). When measured under ear-

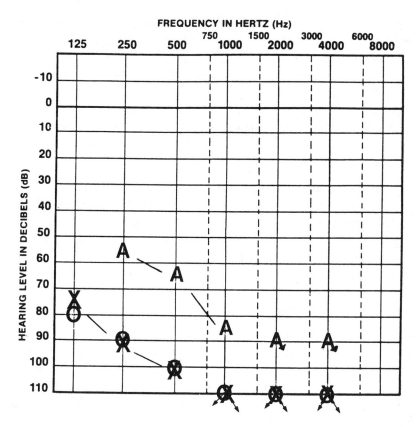

Figure 3–2: An audiogram that indicates the softest sound that can be heard by the child at each pitch (frequency). The left ear thresholds are represented by an "X" and the right ear by an "O." These thresholds were obtained while the child was wearing earphones. In this example, an audiogram is shown for a child with a profound hearing loss. The "A's" indicate the child's thresholds when wearing a hearing aid. Audiometrically, this child is a candidate for a cochlear implant.

phones, pure tones are used as stimuli. When measured in sound field, narrowbands of noise or warble tones are used. The sound field measurements can either be made without an assistive device (unaided) or with a hearing aid, tactile aid, or cochlear implant (aided).

A complete audiogram indicates whether the hearing loss is conductive or sensorineural in nature. A *conductive* loss occurs when there is an obstruction or disease in the external ear canal or in the middle ear. A perforated eardrum or an ear infection resulting in fluid in the middle ear may result in a conductive hearing loss. A *sensorineural* hearing loss indicates that there is a deficit in the sensory cells of the inner ear or the hearing nerve that carries information to the brain. Nearly all types of sensorineural hearing losses can benefit from a hearing aid. Hearing aids are sometimes used for people with conductive hearing losses if the cause of the loss can not be remediated by medical treatment. Cochlear implants are appropriate only for children with a sensorineural hearing loss.

Hearing loss is also classified by the degree of impairment. Five categories are often used to describe the loss and its handicapping effects: mild, moderate, severe, profound, and total. In general, the greater the degree of hearing loss, the greater the loss in understanding speech and the subsequent handicapping effects on oral speech and language development. Cochlear implants are appropriate only for some of the children with severe, profound, or total hearing loss. An audiogram from a child appropriate for a cochlear implant is shown in Figure 3–2.

As well as an indication of the degree and type of hearing loss, the audiogram may provide some information about the person's ability to understand the auditory speech signal. However, it does so only in a general way. For example, those speech sounds, or parts of speech sounds, that are below the child's hearing threshold will not be heard. Figure 3–3 shows an audiogram with the approximate sound levels of different speech sounds superimposed upon it. Most speech sounds contain energy in the entire frequency region, but this simplified graph shows the frequency and intensity regions where the important information is located.

Speech sounds that are above threshold can not always be heard clearly. For example, many speech sounds may be above threshold for a child with a cochlear implant. However, these sounds may be distorted and not be recognizable to the child, even though he can hear them. Thus, great care must be used when viewing and interpreting the audiogram of an implanted child. The best way to determine a child's speech understanding ability is to measure it directly.

speech perception tests

Speech perception testing is fundamental to cochlear implant candidate selection because it is critical to determine how much benefit the child

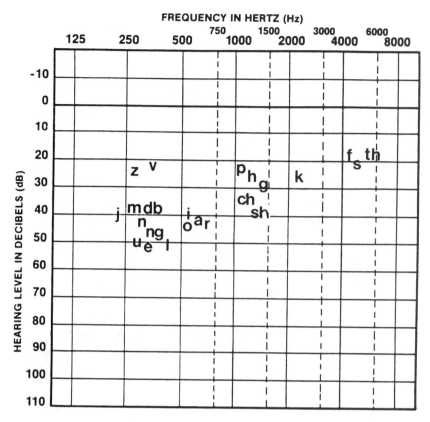

FREQUENCY IN HERTZ (Hz)

Figure 3–3: This audiogram shows the approximate pitch and loudness of many consonants and vowels. If a child's thresholds are poorer than these levels, as would be the case for the child depicted in Figure 3–2, then he will not hear the speech sounds. If a child's thresholds are better than these levels, then the child should detect them. However, just because these sounds are detected does not ensure that they will be understood.

receives from a hearing aid. If a child receives only limited information from his hearing aid, he may be a candidate for a cochlear implant. If he is getting substantial information, then he is not a cochlear implant candidate.

When testing speech perception ability in adults, we often simply present them with a word or sentence, and ask them to repeat what they heard. Testing children is more difficult, because it is necessary to consider their language ability, their cognitive or knowledge level, their

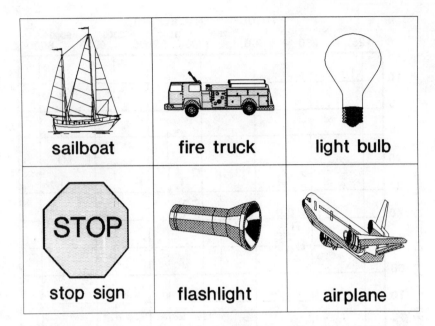

Figure 3–4: An example of a six-choice closed-set test. The child hears one word, and must select from the six choices which one he thinks he hears.

attention span, and vocabulary. Because of all these factors, different tests must be used for children in different age ranges. Some of the tests are similar to the adult tests, only with simpler vocabulary. To make the test easier, often a set of alternative choices are available to the child. Figure 3–4 shows a set of six choices of two syllable words. During testing, the child is presented with one of the words, such as *airplane*, and selects among the six options.

It is often desirable to measure how the implant enhances a child's ability to recognize speech audiovisually. An evaluation of speechreading enhancement compares the child's ability to understand speech by lipreading the talker without sound, to his ability to lipread and listen with his cochlear implant.

Some speech perception tests measure how well the child perceives the gross characteristics of speech, such as loudness changes over time, or differences between voiced and unvoiced sounds (for example, between *bit* and *pit*, or between *save* and *safe*). Some tests focus on the child's ability to hear the different number of syllables in words. For

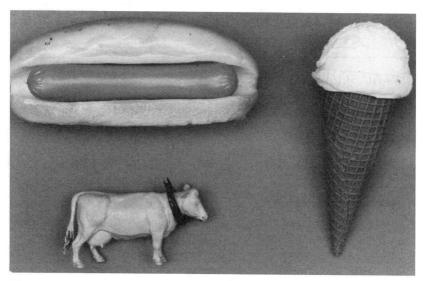

Figure 3–5: An example of a simple closed-set test appropriate for a young child. Its purpose is to determine if the child can identify the item based on the number of syllables.

example, the stimuli shown in Figure 3–5 can be used to measure whether the child can discriminate single syllable words from multi-syllable words. During testing, the audiologist says one of the words. The child's task is to touch the word that he heard. The test is scored by computing how many times the child selected a multisyllable word after hearing a multisyllable word, and how many times he selected a single syllable word after hearing a single syllable word.

Some implant users may not develop the skills to recognize words or sentences, but most are able to recognize the loudness and timing fluctuations of speech. This skill usually enhances their ability to per-ceive speech audiovisually (that is, to speechread).

variables that influence performance

A number of variables can influence how much benefit a child receives from an implant. These factors, listed in Table 3–1, provide some ex-planation for the individual differences observed among children with cochlear implants.

Table 3–1:   Factors That May Influence the Performance of Children with a Cochlear Implant.

VARIABLE	EFFECT
Onset of hearing loss	Individuals with a postlingual hearing loss have a better memory for speech and usually perform better than individuals with a prelingual hearing loss.
Years of deafness	Individuals who have been deaf for a short period of time may perform better than those who have been deaf a long period of time.
Etiology	Diseases that fill the cochlear with bone or destroy hair cells and nerves will inhibit success, but the effects of disease are difficult to determine prior to implantation.
Rehabilitation	Children who obtain systematic aural rehabilitation will likely progress faster than those who do not.
Family support	Children show benefit when their family assists with the care of the implant, facilitates rehabilitation, and provides an environment that is rich with sound.
Age at implantation	It may be better if the child receives the implant sooner than later, provided that he can be tested and found to be an appropriate candidate.
Communication style	Interested communicators may perform better than passive communicators.

prelingual versus postlingual hearing loss

The process of learning language begins at birth. Hearing children develop a memory for the important rules of auditory language during their first two or three years of life. Children who became profoundly deaf after they learned language are *postlingually* deaf. Children who became deaf before they learned language are *prelingually* deaf. Prelingually deaf children who are born deaf are *congenitally* deaf. In many cases it is uncertain when the child became profoundly deaf or how much exposure to spoken language he had prior to acquiring a hearing loss.

Postlingually deaf children have memories of the speech signal and language. They can remember how many words sound. Cochlear implants present imperfect representations of speech. When postlingually deafened children hear the imperfect word with the cochlear implant, they are often able to match it to what they know the word is supposed to sound like.

Prelingually deaf children have no previous memory of speech. Therefore, when they hear the new, somewhat distorted sounds provided by the implant, they must learn to associate labels to them. Many prelingually deafened children are able to do this with the cochlear implant, but it takes much longer for them to achieve this level of performance than it does for postlingually deaf children.

length of deafness

The ability to remember what speech and environmental signals sound like is important for children and adults who use cochlear implants. After people have been deaf for many years, they can forget the sounds of the world. They may also forget the muscle movements and kinesthetic feelings used to produce some sounds, and as a result, their speech production skills may deteriorate. The rate at which children forget the speech sounds varies enormously from one child to another.

Research with postlingually deafened adults with cochlear implants suggest that, in general, adults who have been deaf for several years before receiving a cochlear implant do not perform as well as adults who receive a cochlear implant shortly after becoming deaf. This may be related to the observation that some loss of nerve fibers occurs when the hearing system does not receive stimulation for prolonged periods of time. Even though the benefit may not be as great as for recently deafened users, most postlingually deafened adults benefit from an implant, even after they have been deaf for forty or fifty years.

etiology of deafness

For a cochlear implant to function properly it must be possible to place the array of electrodes adjacent to the remaining hair cells and nerve fibers in the cochlea. There must also be a sufficient number of hair cells and hearing nerve fibers to respond to the electrical stimulation. Any disease process that fills the cochlear duct with bone, or that prevents its normal open development, can impede the placement of electrodes along the cochlear duct. Any disease process that prevents the growth of hair cells or neurons, or that destructs them will interfere with optimal performance with the implant.

Although these disease processes may interfere with optimal performance, as long as the electrode array can be placed adjacent to some surviving nerve fibers, most children will receive some benefit from their cochlear implant. Unfortunately, there are no predictive measures available at this time to determine how many surviving nerve endings exist in a deaf ear before implant surgery.

aural rehabilitation

Aural rehabilitation develops the child's ability to communicate by using hearing (and sometimes vision). A child must learn to use the sounds that are processed by the implant. Since the implant does not restore hearing to normal, the child must learn to recognize distorted sounds. A prelingually deaf child must learn to label these new percepts that are reaching his brain. A postlingually deaf child has an advantage in that he knows what the sounds are supposed to sound like, and will know the grammatical rules of spoken language. However, he will still have to learn to match the sounds produced by the implant to what he has heard in the past.

Some implanted children will spontaneously learn to attend to and interpret sound, but all will require help from parents and teachers to optimize learning. Children who receive daily exposure to speech and regular training in speech and sound recognition will more likely achieve this maximum auditory potential than those children who do not.

There are many different methods for developing a child's ability to understand speech with a cochlear implant. Whatever the particular aural rehabilitation program, a major component of it should include auditory training (Chapter 6). The cochlear implant provides the opportunity for sound to be perceived. It is vitally important that parents and teachers ensure that sound, including speech, is part of the child's environment. Communicative interactions through modalities other than oral speech, such as sign language, are important to maintain if the child is dependent upon them for successful communication. However, some practice in sound and speech recognition should take place everyday to help the child learn to use sound meaningfully.

family support

A child with a cochlear implant will obtain the best results in a nurturing home environment, where all family members support the child's use of the cochlear implant by communicating with him using speech. The family should call the child's attention to meaningful sounds and reinforce his learning. Communication may include sign if he requires it to understand messages. As the child's auditory skills improve, it may be possible to reduce (or eliminate) signing.

The family can also take an active role in ensuring that the cochlear implant is functioning correctly. They must learn how the device works, which of its components can be checked, what can be replaced, and whom to contact to obtain spare parts.

age at implantation

It has been suggested that the younger a child is at the time of implantation, the greater the ultimate benefits will be. At this time, there are no research results directly supporting this theory. However, there does appear to be a critical period for learning language. The literature suggests that normal hearing children need to be exposed to language before the age of about three years for them to develop a language system effortlessly. Similarly, very young children learn a second language more readily than do older children or young adults.

Older adults, in general, do not perform as well with cochlear implants as younger adults. This may be related to the greater adaptiveness of young people to all kinds of stimuli and situations. (It is important to note, however, that many older adults obtain significant benefit from their cochlear implant.)

communication style

The child's personality may affect his use of and ultimate success with the cochlear implant. Our experience suggests that three general categories are appropriate for describing a child's communicative style: **passive, interested, and demanding**. Many variations of each exist, and the same child may exhibit different styles at various times. These categories are described so to facilitate an appreciation of individual differences among children.

The Passive Communicator: The passive communicator is one who rarely requests information. He is not inquisitive about what other people are talking about or listening to. The child may not indicate when he has not understood what has been said to him. Likewise, he may be unwilling to repeat or rephrase a sentence to help a listener understand his speech. The passive communicator tends to lack curiosity about sound in his environment. Adults and children who exhibit these characteristics are often considered "easy-going".

The Interested Communicator: The interested communicator is one who attends to the talker and asks for message clarification when he misunderstands a spoken message. This child often expresses a desire to know what others are talking about even when he is not part of the conversation. An interested communicator shows a natural curiosity about environmental sounds. He takes great pride in communicating with others and is not inhibited about using his voice or sign language. He is often an engaging conversationalist. All other factors equal, the interested communicator will typically show greater gains with an implant than a passive communicator.

The Demanding Communicator: The demanding communicator is an extreme version of the interested communicator. He may have a desire to interact with people and may be curious about what they are saying. However, he ignores the social graces of conversation and may demand information, or become frustrated and agitated when communication breaks down and he is unable to understand or be understood. The child who is a demanding communicator may have other behavioral problems as a result of frustration with communication.

case studies

This section presents the stories of four children who received cochlear implants at the University of Iowa. The case studies were selected to represent different possible outcomes of implantation, and to reflect how patient variables can influence performance.

case study 1: Matthew

Matthew is thought to be congenitally deaf. His mother first suspected he had a hearing loss when he was four months old. After several trips to the pediatrician, a referral was made to an audiologist. When the hearing evaluation was performed at the age of eight months, Matthew's profound hearing loss was confirmed. The cause of his hearing loss was never determined. Within a month after the loss was identified, Matthew was fitted with binaural behind-the-ear hearing aids and his parents began taking sign language classes at the community college.

Matthew received services from an itinerant teacher of the hearing impaired until, at age three years, he entered a pre-school program that utilized total communication. He used his hearing aids on a full time basis, but his parents questioned whether or not they were beneficial.

When Matthew was seen for a cochlear implant evaluation at the age of three years, seven months, he had good expressive and receptive sign skills and was an attentive and interested communicator for his age. Matthew's parents believed that he had never responded to environmental sounds or speech with or without his hearing aids. He had no intelligible speech although he did use his voice when signing, with his parent's prompting.

Matthew received a multichannel cochlear implant at the age of three years, ten months. All the electrodes were placed in the cochlea. At the time of the initial stimulation, Matthew expressed great delight in hearing the soft and loud beeps while the speech processor was being adjusted. However, when the implant microphone was activated, and the audiologist said his name, Matthew became frightened and upset. Several days elapsed before he would wear the implant for more than a few minutes. By gradually increasing the amount of time he wore the implant during the following weeks, Matthew became comfortable with the device. Within two months of the initial stimulation he wore the implant on a full-time basis, at home and at pre-school, without problem.

While Matthew could identify the presence of sound during the initial processor adjustment phase, the concept of "too loud" was difficult for him to internalize. Because of this, the device was set to limit the highest output to conservatively low levels. Six additional processor adjustment sessions were required during the first four months to increase the tolerable loudness output so that the full dynamic range of the device could be utilized.

After six months of implant use, Matthew was babbling and using his voice during almost all waking hours. It became necessary for his parents to initiate a "quiet time" to provide some relief to the household. Matthew would indicate the presence of several household sounds, such as the microwave alarm, the telephone, and the dog barking. He did not respond to his name when called unless he was speechreading the talker.

The results of the speech perception tests completed with Matthew at the six-month post-implant evaluation were not significantly different from the results of the pre-implant evaluation, with one exception. Matthew had much improved sound detection skills. He was using his voice consistently when signing, but his only recognizable words were approximations of *mom*, *fine*, and *bye-bye*.

During the next six months, Matthew's parents reported almost weekly changes in his sound awareness and communication skills. At the time of the twelve-month evaluation, Matthew's repertoire of speech sounds had doubled. While his speech was still unintelligible, he was voicing the correct number of syllables and using a well-modulated voice quality. On tests of speech perception ability, Matthew could easily identify patterns of sounds as well as many environmental sounds from a set of four choices. He could also identify single and two-syllable words from a set of four choices with almost 100 percent accuracy. He responded to his name consistently and would initiate conversations with others. Matthew tried repeatedly to be understood and to understand others.

Over the next year, Matthew's listening and speech production skills would progress rapidly, and then show periods of slow progress. At the time of his last cochlear implant evaluation, Matthew had to be reminded to use sign language when communicating with familiar talkers. His speech was judged to be approximately 25 percent intelligible. He was enrolled in a self-contained hearing-impaired classroom for half of the day and mainstreamed with an interpreter in a regular kindergarten for the rest of the day.

case study 2: Becky

Becky's profound deafness was diagnosed at the age of fourteen months of age. It was thought to be caused by a virus, cytomegalovirus (CMV), that her mother was exposed to during her pregnancy. Becky was fitted with a body aid at the age of eighteen months. According to her parents, she resisted using the hearing aid and showed no sound awareness when it was turned on. She wore the hearing aid inconsistently until she was four years old. At that time, Becky's audiologist provided her with a tactile aid. Becky appeared to respond to sound with the tactile aid, which she used primarily at school. Becky was enrolled in a parent/ infant program for hearing-impaired children until she entered a total communication preschool program for hearing-impaired children at the age of three years. At age five years, she entered the total communication kindergarten program.

Becky was seen for a cochlear implant evaluation at the age of six years. At that time, she communicated almost exclusively with sign language and had to be prompted to use her voice. Her expressive and receptive sign skills were considered average for her age and degree of hearing loss.

Becky underwent cochlear implant surgery at the age of six years, two months. All of the electrodes were placed in her cochlea. At the initial stimulation of her implant, Becky's response to sound was unremarkable. She did not object to wearing the device, but she did not appear curious about or interested in sound. She consistently indicated when sound was present and quickly learned to scale the loudness of sound reliably. Only three tune-up sessions were required to program the speech processor.

By the six-month post-implant evaluation, Becky demonstrated consistent sound awareness when she was placed in a structured listening situation and asked to indicate when she heard a sound. However, Becky did not show awareness to sound in unstructured situations. The results of speech perception testing indicated no significant change in her abilities compared to the pre-implant evaluation. Her speech production skills were unchanged as well. While Becky reportedly wore the implant all during the school day, she typically removed it when she came home and seldom used it on the weekends.

The results of the twelve-month evaluation were not significantly different from the six-month evaluation. Becky was still not using the implant on a full time basis. She began to actively resist wearing the device except when at school and she often left it in her classroom over the weekend. Becky's parents were counseled about the importance of supporting her use of the implant. They were asked to keep a weekly log of her use time and activities were suggested to encourage her to attend to sound.

Over the next year, Becky's use of the implant became more consistent, although she did not wear it all day, every day. She began to hum continuously. She used her voice in play, but she had to be prompted to use it for communication. In order to motivate Becky to improve her speech skills, her speech-language pathologist developed, with Becky's input, a list of functional words that Becky wanted to learn to say. Within a few weeks, Becky could produce some of the words when modeling the therapist. It was reinforcing for Becky when she could successfully produce a word or phrase that her parents and hearing friends could understand. About this time, her reading skills began to improve, and Becky could read aloud to her parents as part of a daily bedtime routine. These activities were also reinforcing to Becky and her parents.

During the next few months, Becky's resistance to the implant decreased, and she began to use it on a full time basis. At the time of her last visit to the implant center, almost two and a half years after her surgery, Becky showed measurable improvement on the speech perception tests. She responded to her name and recognized a number of environmental sounds. Her parents reported that she had shown increasing interest in communicating with others, and was almost completely responsible for handling and taking care of her implant.

case study 3: Karen

Karen's hearing loss was first identified at the age of five years during a kindergarten health screening. At that time, she had a mild sensorineural hearing loss in both ears. She was fitted with bilateral behind-the-ear hearing aids which she wore all waking hours. Over the next six years, audiological tests showed a gradual decrease in Karen's hearing levels. She was fitted with more powerful hearing aids, and learned how to fingerspell. When she experienced difficulty in under-standing her family, they fingerspelled words to her. Karen is a very good lipreader.

By the age of twelve years, Karen had a profound loss bilaterally. She is considered postlingually deaf. The cause of her hearing loss has never been determined. She wore a hearing aid in her left ear when not in school. An auditory trainer was used during the school day. Karen began using an interpreter on a full time basis for her academic classes when she started fifth grade. While her speech skills remained good, her voice quality had become increasingly nasal. She used sign lan-guage and fingerspelling receptively.

Karen underwent surgery to receive a cochlear implant at the age of thirteen years, four months. At the time of the initial stimulation, Karen was immediately able to understand some of the audiologist's speech without lipreading. She found the quality of speech strange, but quickly adapted to full time implant use. With the implant and speechreading, Karen could understand almost all of an informal conversation. She even had limited telephone use.

Over the next six months, Karen wore her implant all waking hours. She resumed all the normal activities of a junior high school student, including playing basketball. Her speech became noticeably less nasal. Her speech perception skills were as good as some of the best implant users tested at the University of Iowa Hospital. She continued to use a full time interpreter for her academic classes, but used sign language only occasionally for receptive communication. At the time of her last implant evaluation, two years after her surgery, Karen's auditory skills were continuing to improve, though less dramatically compared to the first six months of implant use.

case study 4: Anita

Anita became profoundly deaf at the age of five months when she contracted spinal meningitis. Her deafness was diagnosed immediately thereafter. She is considered to be prelingually deaf. She was fitted with binaural behind-the-ear hearing aids at age six months. Her entire family enrolled in sign language classes. Sign language was not totally foreign to the family since Anita's aunt, who had been deaf since birth and lived nearby, used sign in addition to oral speech.

Anita was enrolled in a hearing-impaired preschool program at two years of age. Her speech and signing skills were considered to be very good for such a young child. She was an interested communicator and was always encouraged to use her voice in addition to sign language. Throughout her elementary school years, Anita was mainstreamed with an interpreter and was seen by the teacher of the hearing impaired only for supplemental language and reading help.

When Anita entered junior high school, she began to have some difficulty maintaining her academic progress. She discontinued using an auditory trainer at school but wore her personal hearing aids during all waking hours. She was unable to understand speech or interpret many environmental sounds, but she felt that her hearing aid in the right ear in particular was helpful for speechreading and sound awareness.

Anita was seen for a cochlear implant evaluation at the age of fourteen years. After several assessments and much discussion with her family and teachers, it was determined that Anita might benefit from an implant. She was scheduled for cochlear implant surgery for her left ear.

At the initial stimulation of the implant, Anita did not experience a sensation of hearing. Instead, she reported vibration in her head and shoulders when sound was presented. After using the implant for several weeks, she reported that the sensations became less tactile and more sound-like. After using the processor at school and at home for several months, Anita could identify many environmental sounds; for example, the telephone and the doorbell ringing. She continued to use her hearing aid in the right ear. She was disappointed that she could not understand speech with the implant nor use the telephone to talk to her friends.

Six months after the initial stimulation, Anita's speech perception test results were not significantly different compared to the results before surgery when she used her hearing aids. Her parents reported that she had begun to use the implant less and had to be reminded to take it to school with her. Despite much support and encouragement from her friends and family, Anita felt discouraged. She claimed she disliked wearing the speech processor because it interfered with her movement and she did not like the way it looked. Several attempts were made by her parents to reinforce Anita for using the implant. However, after several months of arguing, they decided to let her make the decision to discontinue using it.

When contacted a year after Anita's surgery date, her parents reported that Anita would occasionally wear her implant at home and when she babysat a neighbor's child. Her parents believed that Anita might decide to wear the implant more in the future, but that it would be her choice to do so.

summary

In this chapter we have discussed the variables that affect hearing abilities of children with cochlear implants. Hearing abilities can be measured in several ways. The audiogram is a measurement of the softest sounds the child can detect, but it does not indicate the child's ability to understand speech. For this, a variety of speech perception tests can be used, including audiovisual tests that measure speech-reading enhancement.

A variety of factors contribute to a child's ability to understand speech with a cochlear implant. Postlingually deafened children typically perform better than prelingually deafened children, because they remember speech sounds and often have a greater knowledge of English. Children tend to perform better if they have been deaf for a short time, if they receive aural rehabilitation, if the family plays an active role and provides a rich sound environment, if they are young, and if they are active communicators.

references

Tyler, R.S., Berliner, K., Demorest, M., Hirshorn, M., Luxford, W., and Mangham, C. (1986). Clinical objectives and research-design issues for cochlear implants in children. *Seminars in Hearing*, 7(4), 433–440.

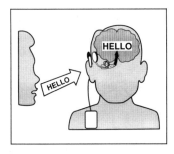

4

conversing with the
implanted child
nancy tye-murray, ph.d.

Most children have a communication mode in place prior to receiving an implant. The cochlear implant need not alter it. However,
once the child is wearing his device on a regular basis, he should attempt
to communicate aurally/orally for part of each day, regardless of how
he communicates most frequently. Hearing must become a part of the
child's personality and self image if he is to benefit from wearing an
implant.

This chapter describes the communication modes that are used by deaf
children, and considers how an implant will affect communication style.
It then reviews techniques for engaging the child in conversation. Finally,
talker behaviors and room acoustics that can promote successful aural/
oral communication are considered.

communication modes

There are a number of different communication modes that individuals
with profound hearing impairment may use. They fall along a continuum,

from being exclusively manual to being aural/oral. Four general communication modes are described here, beginning with American Sign
Language, which is a manual system.

American Sign Language

American Sign Language (ASL) is the most commonly used manual
language in North America. Its grammar differs from that of spoken
English. For instance, some ASL signs represent a concept or state of
being rather than a single word. Many function words, such as pronouns
and articles, are indicated by body and facial movements and are not
signed separately. The child who uses ASL does not attempt to speak
and sign simultaneously.

Because the grammar of ASL does not correspond to spoken English,
it is not used in most primary level educational settings, where children
learn to read and write. Most children with hearing parents (about 90
percent of all severely and profoundly hearing-impaired children) learn
ASL from hearing-impaired friends and hearing-impaired adults in late
childhood or early adulthood.

Although few implanted children use ASL, it might become more prev-
alent in the future. A number of speech and hearing professionals and
members of the deaf community advocate that ASL be adopted in the
public school systems (Lane, 1984; Johnson, Liddell, & Erting, 1989).
They suggest that severely and profoundly hearing-impaired children
who communicate with ASL may develop cognitive skills and learn
academic material more easily than children who communicate with an
English-based language system.

total communication

Total communication combines manually coded English with oral speech.
Signs corresponding to words are presented in the same word order
as English. The talker speaks and simultaneously signs the message.
The child uses every available avenue to perceive the message, including sign, lipreading, and residual hearing. The child also learns to
attend to nonlinguistic cues, such as facial expressions and hand gestures.

cued speech

Cued speech uses phonemically-based hand gestures to supplement speechreading (Cornett, 1967). Eight different handshapes distinguish consonants that look alike on the mouth. For instance, the consonants /p/ (as in *pea*) and /b/ (*bee*) look alike. The consonant /p/ is shown by a 1 handshape and /b/ is shown by a 4 handshape. Vowels that look alike on the mouth are distinguished with six hand positions. For instance, the vowels /i/ (*pea*) and /e/ (*pay*) look alike. The vowel /i/ is represented by a handshape at the throat and /e/ is represented by a handshape on the chin. A talker saying the word *pea* would hold a 1 handshape to the throat as he or she simultaneously said the word.

Not many deaf and hearing-impaired children use cued speech at present, although the system is growing in popularity.

aural/oral communication

When two individuals communicate in an aural/oral mode, the talker speaks and the receiver attends to the audiovisual or auditory-only speech signal. Most children who communicate aurally/orally and receive a cochlear implant have a postlingual hearing loss. This is because a prelingual and profound hearing loss prevents most individuals from learning a language system aurally/orally.

using a communication mode with an implanted child

It is vital that the child has abundant auditory speech stimulation after receiving a cochlear implant, and that he begin to rely on the speech signal for communication. A child's awareness of and reliance on the speech signal can be nurtured within the domains of his particular communication mode.

ASL

Individuals should not speak when using ASL or else the grammar of both their ASL message and their spoken message will become distorted. It is very difficult to use ASL and an English-based system, or any two language systems, simultaneously. This truism suggests that if a child communicates exclusively with ASL, he will not learn to utilize the information provided by his cochlear implant. He will seldom hear his own speech or that of others.

An implanted child who communicates with ASL must learn the language of spoken English through speechreading, listening, and reading. The child should attempt to communicate aurally/orally for part of each day. If a teacher is in an ASL classroom, she should often talk rather than sign to the child when interacting on a one-on-one basis. If there is a classroom aid with normal hearing, the child should have daily opportunity to interact aurally/orally with this individual. The child might attend a hearing classroom for nonacademic subjects such as art, where he can attempt aural/oral communication. He should receive much speechreading training, and after acquiring some experience with the device, auditory training.

total communication

Parents and teachers must revise their perception of their child after he receives an implant; he is now an individual with some hearing potential. Many parents and teachers have inconsistently used voice when using total communication, assuming that their child could not hear. They must begin talking aloud, with words that match their signs. The child will only learn to attend to and interpret the speech signal if he hears it often. The child should receive both speechreading and auditory training.

Most implanted children who used total communication prior to implantation will always depend on sign to some degree and many will never develop the skills to communicate without it. The family and the child, the age of the child at implantation, and the benefit afforded by the cochlear implant will determine what communication system is used most often. However, the child should attempt to communicate with an aural/oral mode for at least a part of each day.

aural/oral communication and cued speech

The cochlear implant should not affect how the parent or teacher and the child interact when using aural/oral communication, other than to facilitate communication. The child must learn to associate the new auditory signal with speech, and will benefit from an increased amount of auditory training. If the child uses cued speech, he should speechread without hand cues daily.

Table 4–1: Guidelines for Conversing with an Implanted Child.

> **A.** Initialize the conversation.
> **B.** Organize the message.
> **C.** Encourage the child's participation.
> **D.** Establish comprehension.
> **E.** Repair breakdowns in communication.

talking with an implanted child using an aural/oral mode

Conversational interactions are the most effective means to develop an implanted child's ability to perceive speech. Conversing aurally/orally with an implanted child may be a novel experience for some parents and teachers if prior to implantation they used only manual communication.

This section provides guidelines for conversing aurally/orally with the implanted child. The guidelines are listed in Table 4–1. An aural/oral interaction may only last a few minutes and may occur only once or twice a day. Following these guidelines may make the interaction a positive experience for both child and parent or teacher.

attract the child's attention

Before beginning an aural/oral conversation, the parent or teacher must attract the child's attention (Table 4–2). She can say his name or gently touch his shoulder. She might use, a hand or head gesture to indicate her topic of conversation. For instance, a teacher might look at her watch before saying, "Time to go home."

The talker should establish eye contact prior to speaking so that the child will not miss the beginning of her utterance, and so that he can better speechread her. The best topics for conversation are those that interest the child.

A parent or teacher can initiate a conversation by attending to the child's mood, actions, and gaze. If the child looks toward an apple, she can remark about the apple. If he pushes a toy airplane, she can comment

Table 4–2: Ways to Attract the Child's Attention During Aural/Oral Communication.

A. Say the child's name or gently touch his shoulder.

B. Establish the topic of conversation.

C. Vary vocal intensity.

D. Vary intonation.

E. Establish eye contact.

F. Spark the child's interest.

G. Be attentive to the child's moods, actions, and gaze.

---

about the flying plane. In one language session, a child and his teacher were playing with clay. The child seemed disinterested and unresponsive. When he half-heartedly attempted to roll the clay, the teacher looked impressed. "You made someone's head", she said. The child responded by adding more clay, and then looked at the teacher for a reaction. By responding to the child's mood and actions, the teacher had created a starting point for conversation.

organize the message

People communicate messages by speaking a series of related sentences; rarely do they speak sentences in isolation. A well-organized message will be easier for the child to understand than one that is poorly organized. In fact, sometimes implanted children will misperceive utterances because they are not well-organized, and not because of their limited perceptual skills. Principles of good message organization are listed in Table 4–3.

Creating an organized message does not require special talent or great effort. The talker can present organized messages by taking time to think and plan before speaking, by speaking slowly, and by learning to monitor her own utterances (that is, by listening to herself as she talks).

engage the child

Whenever they communicate aurally/orally, the teacher or parent should encourage the child to be an active rather than passive conversational

Table 4-3: Organize the Message Before Talking to the Child.

A. Provide adequate information. Not enough information will confuse the child; too much will lose his interest or confuse him.

B. Present information sequentially. A narrative has a beginning, a middle, and a conclusion. An activity consists of a series of steps or directions; for example, *First you. . . .Then you. . . .Finally you. . . .*

C. Use precise language and avoid ambiguity. For instance, the sentence, *Your jeans are in the drawer*, is more precise and less ambiguous than, *They are over there.*

D. Do not use convoluted syntax and semantics. The sentence, *The blue jeans are in the drawer*, is more appropriate than, *The blue jeans, which you can wear with the red sweater, are in the bottom drawer over there.*

E. Avoid telegraphic speech. An utterance such as, *Wear red sweater.*, is unacceptale.

---

partner. If the child helps to maintain and shape the conversation, he will be more motivated to converse and more motivated to attend to the speech signal. Three types of communication acts can be used to engage the child in conversation: questions, comments, and acknowlegements.

Questions: Questions require a response from the child. They can be of the two-choice type:

> Are you happy?
>
> Do you want the small or large one?

Questions can also be of the **wh-type**:

> Who is that?
>
> Where are you going?
>
> What did you say?
>
> Why are you taking the shoes?
>
> When is the appointment?
>
> Which one do you want?

Questions can initiate a conversation. The talker might ask, "What's that?", or, "What are you doing?". Questions can also maintain a conversation. For instance, the child might be telling a story using total communication. The talker can ask without sign, "And then what happened?" If they are coloring, she might ask, "What should I draw now?"

A child needs time to answer a question that is presented aurally/orally. If he does not respond immediately, the talker should not assume that he did not understand it. She should pause for an ample time period before repeating or restructuring the question, or before answering it herself. The child is developing his perceptual abilities and his language and discourse skills; he must recognize what information is required and then formulate a reply.

There is a danger in asking too many questions. A conversation can degenerate into a question-answer session with the parent or teacher asking a series of questions and the child passively responding, often with one- and two-word utterances.

Comments: A comment describes what the parent or teacher or the child is doing or thinking, and may present new information. The talker can express an opinion, speculate, inform, or agree or disagree. When talkers limit the number of questions and use comments, hearing-impaired children become more active conversationalists (Wood, Wood, Griffiths, & Howarth, 1986).

The teacher below uses comments to engage the child:

> **Teacher:** "You are drawing a house."
>
> **Jim:** "Uh-huh."
>
> **Teacher:** "I wonder who lives in the house, maybe a girl."
>
> **Jim:** "A boy! and a dog."
>
> **Teacher:** "Oh, I like dogs."
>
> **Jim:** "A big dog! Jakko!"

In this example, the teacher seems genuinely interested in what the child says. She expresses her opinion (she like dogs) and she speculates about the house's occupant. These contributions of new information provide an opportunity for Jim to take charge and they maintain his interest. Jim responds to the teacher's comments by also offering new information.

The interaction below shows what might have happened if the teacher had asked only questions:

> **Teacher:** "What are you drawing?"
>
> **Jim:** "A house."
>
> **Teacher:** "Who lives in the house?"
>
> **Jim:** "A boy."
>
> **Teacher:** "Does he have a dog?"
>
> **Jim:** "Yes."

In comparison with the previous example, this conversation is an unsatisfactory interaction for both the teacher and Jim. The teacher has complete responsibility for maintaining the conversation; Jim has no control over its direction.

Teachers and parents need not completely avoid using questions when using aural/oral communication, but should limit their number. Children are more likely to be active participants when their conversational partners use comments.

Acknowledgments: Acknowledgments are a form of comment. The parent or teacher may nod her head as the child speaks, and say, "yes . . . uh-huh". She might repeat his utterance. For instance, the child might say, "My truck broke." The teacher might respond, "You broke your truck." Acknowledgments also include exclamations, such as, *Oh, my!, Good job!,* and *Oh boy!.*

Although acknowledgments present no new information, they let the child know that the parent or teacher is listening and that she understands his message. Acknowledgments tell the child that he is interesting and that what he has to say is worth hearing.

establish comprehension

The implanted child will rarely comprehend everything the talker says orally. The talker must use her own judgment to determine whether and when she should repair a breakdown in communication. Certainly if the child is frustrated by not knowing the message, or if it is important that he understand it, the talker should attempt to repair a breakdown.

A child often presents identifiable clues to indicate comprehension. He may follow the talker's command, respond to a comment or question

Table 4–4: Repair Strategies That a Talker Can Use to Rectify a Communication Breakdown.

A. Repetition

B. Simplification
   1. Fewer words
   2. More commonplace words

C. Rephrasing
   1. More visible words
   2. Words that are better specified by context

D. Elaboration
   1. More information
   2. Repeated keywords

E. Keyword

F. Delimiting (closed response set)

G. Building from the known

H. Total communication

---

appropriately, express interest, or respond with an appropriate facial expression or gesture (Adam, Fortier, Schiel, Smith, Soland, & Stone, 1990). When he does not understand, he may look puzzled or anxious, he may seem inattentive, or he may become angry. Frequently the child will bluff; for example, he may nod his head, smile vaguely, or say, "yes . . . uh-huh."

repair breakdowns in communication

The talker can use verbal repair strategies when the child does not understand a spoken message. They require patience and work on the part of the talker, but they can promote successful aural/oral communication. Table 4–4 lists eight repair strategies.

Repeat: The most obvious tact to take when a child misunderstands something is to say it again. Teachers often repeat misperceived messages in the classroom (Erber & Greer, 1973) and repetitions appear to remedy some communication breakdowns (Tye-Murray, Purdy, Woodworth, & Tyler, 1990). However, the talker should not over-use

Table 4–5: Examples of the Simplify-Repair Strategy.

A. Simplifying by using fewer words

Sentence: Your spoon fell on the floor.
Simplification: Your spoon fell.

Sentence: Please write your name on your paper.
Simplification: Write your name.

Sentence: You have ten minutes to work the problems.
Simplification: You have ten minutes.

B. Simplifying by using more commonplace words

Sentence: The daffodil blooms in the spring.
Simplification: The flower blooms in the spring.

Question: Where are my trousers?
Simplification: Where are my pants?

Sentence: The temperature is high.
Simplification: It is hot.

---

this strategy. If the child has not understood any part of the message, it may be as incomprehensible the second time around as it was the first time (Berger, 1972; Gagne & Wyllie, 1990; Kelsay, Tye-Murray, submitted).

Simplify: In the conversation below, the mother repairs aural/oral communication breakdown by simplifying her utterance:

> **Mother:** "Please go to the pantry and get the shears."
>
> **John:** (no response)
>
> **Mother:** "Please get the scissors."

The talker can simplify an utterance by reducing the number of words and by using less complex sentence structures. The talker can also simplify an utterance by using more commonplace words. For instance, the word *scissors* occurs more commonly in everyday conversation than does the word *shears*. The child is more likely to be familiar with *scissors,* and should recognize it more easily.

Table 4–6:   Examples of the Rephrase-Repair Strategy.

A. Rephrasing by using more visible words

Sentence: Read your handout.
Rephrasing: Look at your paper.

Sentence: Would you like a soda?
Rephrasing: Do you want some pop?

Sentence: Eat your carrots.
Rephrasing: Finish your vegetables.

B. Rephrasing by exploiting context

Sentence: We have some cereal.
Rephrasing: We have some cornflakes.

Sentence: Mom fixed breakfast.
Rephrasing: Mom made some pancakes.

Question: Did you do your homework?
Rephrasing: Did you finish you arithmetic?

The talker must never simplify an utterance by using telegraphic speech. For instance, *Get scissors* is an unacceptable simplification. Examples of simplified sentences appear in Table 4–5.

Rephrase: A talker might rephrase the sentence, *The plant is on that counter*, as, *The cactus is by the sink*. A talker can rephrase by using words that are better specified by previous conversation or that appear more visible on the lips. For instance, if the parent and child are repotting a cactus, the word *cactus* might be easier to perceive than the word *plant*. If not, *plant* may be more appropriate because it is more visible. Table 4–6 presents examples of rephrased sentences.

Elaborate: In the aural/oral conversation below, the mother uses the elaborate repair strategy:

Mother: "Do you want some lemonade?"

John: "Huh?"

Mother: "I am thirsty. I want some lemonade. Would you like some lemonade?"

Table 4–7:   Examples of the Elaborate Repair Strategy.

A. Elaborating by providing more information

Sentence: I have my books.
Elaboration: My books are in my backpack.

Sentence: Recess is over.
Elaboration: The bell rang. Recess is over.

Sentence: Let's play baseball.
Elaboration: I have a bat and ball. Let's play baseball.

B. Elaborating by providing more information and repeating keywords

Sentence: The milk is on the table.
Elaboration: I need the milk. The milk is on the table.

Sentence: It's time for lunch.
Elaboration: It's time for lunch. We are having sandwiches for lunch.

Sentence: Put your jacket on.
Elaboration: Your jacket is in the closet. Put your jacket on.

When elaborating a message, the talker provides additional information and may repeat keywords more than once. For instance, the mother notes that she is thirsty and says the word *lemonade* twice. Table 4–7 presents examples of the **elaborate** strategy.

Keyword: Saying an important keyword provides sentence topic and establishes a context for perceiving other words in the sentence. For instance, a talker might repeat the words, *potting soil*, after the child misperceives the sentence, *I need the potting soil*. The talker can supplement the keyword with a gesture; for example, pointing toward the potting soil. Table 4–8 presents examples of the **keyword** strategy.

Delimit: The delimit repair strategy is appropriate when the child misperceives a question:

Mother: "Where should we put the plant?"

John: (no response)

Mother: "Should we put the plant in the sun porch?"

Table 4–8:   Examples of the Keywords Repair Strategy.

Sentence: It's time to go to the library.
Keyword: Library. It's time to go to the library.

Sentence: I'm going shopping.
Keyword: Shopping. I'm going shopping.

Sentence: We'll take the balloons to the party.
Keyword: Balloons. We'll take the balloons.

In this example, the mother limits the child's possible responses to a closed set, *yes* or *no*. The danger in using this strategy is that it can create an illusion that a communication breakdown has been repaired. The child may nod his head, even if he has not understood the question. One way to prevent this from happening is to pose the question in an *either/or* form rather than a *yes/no* form. For instance, the mother might have asked, "Should we put the plant in the porch or the kitchen?" The child must understand the question to respond. Examples of the **delimit** repair strategy appear in Table 4–9.

Build from the Known: In the communication breakdown that occurs below, John may have misunderstood his mother because he could not speechread her request or he may be unfamiliar with the word *pack*:

   Mother: "Pack the potting soil into the pot."

Table 4–9:   Examples of the Delimit-Repair Strategy.

Question: What did you do in school today?
Delimited question: Did you play volleyball or baseball?

Question: Where are you going?
Delimited question: Are you going downstairs or outside?

Question: Whom did you sit with?
Delimited question: Did you sit with Jan or Beth?

Question: What's your favorite color?
Delimited question: Do you like blue or red?

Table 4–10: Examples of the Building from the Known Repair Strategy.

Sentence: Get a drink from the water cooler.
Building from the known: That is a water cooler.
You can get a drink.
Get a drink from the water cooler.

Sentence: Stuff the cotton into the sock.
Building from the known: Here is the cotton.
Here is a sock.
Stuff the cotton into the sock.

Sentence: I see the boat on the horizon.
Building from the known: There's a boat.
The boat is far away.
The boat is on the horizon.

Sentence: Bat the volleyball over the net.
Building from the known: Toss the ball.
Hit the ball with your hand.
Bat the ball over the net.

John: "The pot?"

Mother: "Here is the spoon. Here is the potting soil. Pack the soil into the pot." (She hands him the pot.)

The mother repaired the communication breakdown by building from the known. Given the spoon, the potting soil, and the pot, her son can likely deduce that *pack the potting soil* means *put the soil into the pot*. This strategy expands the child's vocabulary as well as rectifies breakdowns in communication. It is similar to the elaborate repair strategy. Examples of the **building from the known** repair strategy appear in Table 4–10.

Total Communication: The parent or teacher can rectify a communication breakdown by supplementing the spoken message with sign. However, if the communication breakdown occurs when the child is attempting to communicate aurally/orally, she should first use one of the repair strategies described above. This gives the child a second chance to perceive the message audiovisually, and the child learns that misunderstandings can be corrected with speech.

**Table 4–11: Appropriate Talker Behaviors for Communicating
in an Aural/Oral Mode.**

A. Do not obscure your mouth with your hand or other object.

B. Speak slightly more slowly than usual.

C. Articulate words but do not exaggerate oral movements.

D. Use your voice; speak at a normal conversational level or a slightly louder than normal level.

E. Do not shout.

F. Do not speak in profile or from behind the child.

G. Use appropriate facial expressions and hand gestures.

H. Indicate topic changes, either by pausing or with a hand gesture.

I. Vary intonation.

J. Keep your head fairly still.

K. Try not to speak in the presence of background noise or when someone else is speaking.

---

talker behaviors and room acoustics

The talker can facilitate a child's ability to converse aurally/orally by using appropriate speaking behaviors and by ensuring that the environment is not noisy or reverberant. Table 4–11 lists behaviors that a talker can use to promote the child's ability to speechread her. Common sources of reverberation and background noise are presented in Table 4–12.

Room reverberation refers to the repeated reflection of sound against hard surfaces. Reverberated sound interferes with the child's ability to attend to speech. As the speech signal reflects from hard surfaces, it masks ongoing speech. For instance, the reverberant /i/ in *seat* may mask the /t/ as the teacher says, "Please take your seat." Rooms can be acoustically treated to minimize reverberation. Acoustical tile, padded carpeting, drapes, and small fiberglass panels at various locations will absorb reverberant sound (Berg, 1987).

Background noise is any auditory signal that interferes with a child's

Table 4–12: Common Sources of Background Noise and Reverberation.

A. Sources of background noise:
- Television
- Radio
- Other people talking
- Equipment, such as an overhead projector or computer
- Air conditioner or furnace
- Classroom activities, such as rustling paper, moving chairs, and dropping books
- Open windows
- Open classroom doorways
- Kitchen activities, such as an electric appliance, the oven fan, running water, and the dish washer

B. Sources of reverberation:
- Hard walls
- Hard floors
- High ceilings
- Parallel walls
- Reflective windows

---

ability to attend to a talker. A cochlear implant will transmit both the speech signal and background noise in the listening environment.

At school, classroom windows and doors can be kept shut, and a *no-noise* policy established in the hallways to minimize background noise. Noisy film projectors or overhead projectors can be replaced. If the floor is not carpeted, rubber caps can be placed on the legs of chairs and tables (Sanders, 1982). In the home, the television and radio can be turned off or used with low volume settings.

summary

A primary goal for a child who receives a cochlear implant is to develop his skills to converse aurally/orally, at least occasionally. For many children, these skills will emerge slowly. The child may continue to rely upon a manual communication mode, but a new emphasis must be placed upon attending to the audiovisual and auditory speech signals.

The parent or teacher can play a significant role in developing the child's conversational skills, and in ensuring positive conversational experiences. She can attract his attention before speaking and present him with well-organized messages. She can engage him in conversation by using questions, comments, and acknowledgements. The talker can rectify breakdowns in communication by using repair strategies. Repair strategies include repeating an utterance, simplifying it, rephrasing it, elaborating the message, speaking a keyword, delimiting, and building from the known. Finally, the talker can speak with behaviors that promote aural/oral communication, and she can optimize the listening environment.

references

Adam, A.J., Fortier, P., Schiel, G., Smith, M., Soland, C., & Stone, P. (1990). *Listening to Learn: A Handbook for Parents with Hearing-impaired Children.* Washington, D.C.: Alexander Graham Bell Association for the Deaf, Inc.

Berg, F.S. (1987). *Facilitating Classroom Listening: A Handbook for Teachers of Normal and Hard-of-Hearing Students.* Boston, MA: College Hill Press.

Cornett, R.O. (1967). Cued speech. *American Annals of the Deaf, 112,* 3–13.

Erber, N.P. & Greer, C.W. (1973). Communication strategies used by teachers at an oral school for the deaf. *Volta Review, 75,* 480–485.

Gagne, J.P., & Wyllie, K.A. (1989). Relative effectiveness of three repair strategies on the visual-identification of misperceived words. *Ear & Hearing, 10,* 368–374.

Johnson, R.E., Liddell, S.K., & Erting, C.J. (1989). *Unlocking the Curriculum: Principles for Achieving Access in Deaf Education.* Gallaudet Research Institute Working Paper *89-3,* Gallaudet University, Washington, D.C.

Kelsay, D. & Tye-Murray, N. (Submitted). *Communication Strategies Used by Parents of Young Cochlear Implant Recipients.*

Lane, H. (1984). *When the Mind Hears.* New York, NY: Random House.

Sanders, D.A. (1982). *Aural Rehabilitation: A Management View (Second edition).* Englewood Cliffs, NJ: Prentice-Hall.

Tye-Murray, N., Purdy, S.C., Woodworth, G.G., & Tyler, R.S. (1990). Effects of repair strategies on visual identification of sentences. *Journal of Speech and Hearing Disorders, 55,* 621–627.

Wood, D., Wood, H. Griffiths, A., & Howarth, I. (1986). *Teaching and Talking with Deaf Children.* New York, NY: John Wiley & Sons.

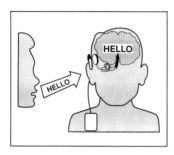

5

teaching speech perception skills: general guidelines

nancy tye-murray, ph.d.

Speech perception training has two components, auditory and speechreading training. The first component develops the implanted child's ability to recognize speech auditorily. The second develops his ability to recognize speech using both audition and vision.

This chapter presents general guidelines for informally and formally developing the implanted child's speech perception skills. Specific guidelines for auditory and speechreading training are presented in Chapters 6 and 7, respectively.

description of speech perception training

Historically, there are two types of speech perception training, *analytic* and *synthetic*. Most speech perception programs include both types.

Analytic instruction focuses the child's attention on recognizing individual speech sounds and syllables. For instance, the child might practice listening to nonsense syllables such as *poe* and isolated words such as *pat* and *pot*. Learning to recognize speech sounds such as /p/ should enhance the child's ability to understand sentence materials.

Synthetic instruction focuses the child's attention on recognizing the general idea of the message. For instance, the teacher might expect the child to answer a question, even though he may not have understood every word.

Speech perception training may be formal or informal. Training may occur during designated periods of the day and include drill exercises. For instance, the teacher and child might sit at a table. The teacher speaks a series of words and sentences and asks the child to repeat them. This kind of training is referred to as *formal*. Alternatively, the teacher may try to incorporate speech perception practice into other activities. For instance, she might often omit signing as she explains how to construct a puppet during art class. This type of training is referred to as *informal*.

speech perception training in the schools

Training that occurs in the school system must be scheduled around other academic subjects and school activities. As a result, most cochlear implant recipients receive relatively little formal instruction.

Teachers of twelve children who received cochlear implants at the University of Iowa Hospitals and Clinics completed a questionnaire to address three issues: a) how much auditory training and speechreading training occurs in the school setting, b) whether implanted children perform similar types of training activities as their hearing-impaired classmates, and c) whether training occurs in group or individual sessions and whether recorded or live-voice stimuli are used.

The implanted children attended self-contained classrooms for hearing-impaired children and used total communication as their primary mode of communication.

The results indicated that implanted and hearing-impaired classmates received the same amount of speechreading training at school; an average of half an hour per week. Both groups received about one hundred and thirty minutes of auditory training weekly. With one exception, the teachers reported that they used the same type of speech perception training activities with their implanted student as with the other hearing-impaired students. Training typically occurred in group sessions (85 percent of the time) with live-voice stimuli.

auditory training versus speechreading training

Given the limited time available for speech perception training, the teacher must often decide whether to provide auditory or speechreading training to the implanted child, or a little of both. Unfortunately, there are no clear-cut guidelines for making this decision. With some exceptions, we recommend that children receive an equal amount of both types of training. A child with minimal speech recognition skills, limited language, and a congenital hearing loss should receive more speechreading training initially than auditory training. A child with good speechreading abilities and a postlingual hearing loss should receive more auditory training.

In order to develop his auditory skills, the child must occasionally rely only on the auditory signal for understanding spoken messages. Auditory training is valuable because it attunes the implanted child to the presence of sound. It helps the child associate the speech signal with sign vocabulary and with the communication process, and teaches him to recognize speech. It may also influence his speech production skills.

Speechreading training is also valuable and should not be neglected. Prior to receiving an implant, the child perceived speech as a visual event. He now must learn to associate visual articulatory movements with the corresponding auditory signal. Most implant users recognize more speech when they can hear and see the talker than when they only hear the signal. Since the primary goal of perception training is to maximize the child's ability to comprehend speech, the modality that permits the best reception of this information, audiovisual, should often be used during training.

informal speech perception training

Whenever possible, speech perception training should be fun and informal. Younger children should not regard it as work, especially when at home. Training for children who are implanted at an older age may have to be more formal since they may not learn to use the auditory signal as quickly.

In providing informal speech perception training, parents and teachers can occasionally omit signing during familiar routines and when talking about the here and now. They can establish a context using sign before requesting the child to speechread. They can also create opportunities for the child to converse aurally/orally with other children. This section describes these four methods for providing informal speech perception training.

familiar routines

A parent or teacher should try to use less sign during routine or ritual activities. For instance, one implanted child had a well-established bed-time routine. Her father would say without sign, "Time to brush your teeth. Here's the toothbrush. Here's the toothpaste." The child understood her father's message, even though she did not recognize his every word.

Using speech to communicate is natural when the parent and child are working together in the kitchen. Vocabulary and sentences can relate to objects that the parent is manipulating, such as a mixer or spatula, so to provide context cues for the child as he speechreads. The parent might say and sign, "My hands are busy. Please try to speechread me." Table 5–1 presents a list of other familiar routines that present opportunities for aural/oral communication.

the here and now

When initially speaking without sign, the talker should limit conversation to the here and now. The talker can speak about things that she or the child are doing or about objects in the environment. The child will not understand her if she talks about events in the past or about plans for the future. For instance, the child will not recognize a sentence such as, *We're going to the mall on Thursday night*, if he is getting ready for school in the morning.

The parent or teacher can provide a commentary as she performs a particular activity, even though the child seems to understand only part of what she says. For instance, a mother might describe each step in

Table 5–1: **Activities That Present Opportunities for Aural/Oral Communication.**

Communication opportunities include:
- Getting ready for bed,
- Getting dressed in the morning,
- Making cookies,
- Putting toys away,
- Feeding a pet,
- Playing cards,
- Coloring pictures,
- Getting ready for recess,
- Getting ready to go home from school,
- Doing the laundry,
- Setting the table,
- Cleaning the kitchen.

---

doing the laundry. Over time, the context of the setting will give meaning to her words (Ling, 1988).

established context

If the child typically uses total communication, the talker can use sign and speech to establish a context for subsequent aural/oral communication. The talker can tell a story, verbally paint a scene, or speculate about what a classmate or parent is doing. Once the stage has been set, the talker can continue without sign.

The exchange below presents an example of establishing context:

> **Mother:** (with sign and speech) "Your father went to the grocery store. I hope he buys some milk."
>
> **Jean:** (with sign and speech) "I want chocolate."
>
> **Mother:** (with speech only) "I asked him to buy chocolate milk."

creating opportunities for aural/oral communication

One means of developing aural/oral skills is to ensure that the child interacts with normal hearing children. Ling (1988) recommends that parents obtain outdoor equipment such as swing sets and slides to attract a neighborhood friend to the home. For older implant recipients, a basketball hoop, a volleyball net, and computer games that require two participants are appropriate.

Enrolling the child in sports and after-school groups will promote interactions with normal hearing children. Whenever possible, the parent should capitalize on the child's interests, such as arts and crafts or Scouts.

(Even though implanted children should increase their interactions with normal hearing friends, they should be encouraged to maintain friendships with hearing-impaired children and other implant users. These latter friendships will enhance their emotional and social growth, and help them develop a positive self image.)

formal speech perception training

Formal speech perception training for implanted children need not differ qualitatively from that which is provided to severely hearing-impaired children who wear hearing aids. The same training materials can be used with both populations. When the child first receives his implant, he may perform more poorly than the severely hearing-impaired child. Ultimately, he may develop superior skills. Teachers must always be cognizant of a child's progress, and never underestimate his abilities. The implanted child should perhaps receive *more* speech perception practice than the hearing-impaired child; the child with a cochlear implant must learn to use new auditory information whereas the hearing-impaired child typically has adapted to having residual hearing.

training materials and activities

Materials and activities must be appropriate for the child's language skills. They should present familiar linguistic structures and vocabulary. The training materials should relate to the child's everyday experiences. If he practices recognizing sentences, they might relate to a science or math class, or relate to a particular interest such as soccer.

Training activities should present words, phrases, and sentences by a variety of talkers (including children), particularly after the first year of implant use. For instance, /b/ might be presented in several syllable contexts, such as *beet*, *boot*, and *bat*, each spoken by a different talker or several different talkers (possibly using video and/or audio tape). In this way, the child learns that /b/ is the same sound whether it is spoken by a male or female, and regardless of vowel context. Through repeated exposure to different talkers and different contexts, the child learns to abstract what makes a sound or word unique from other sounds and words (Tye-Murray, Tyler, Lansing, & Bertschy, 1990). This is how normal hearing infants develop speech listening skills.

The materials should be designed so that they challenge the child, but also allow him to experience success frequently. Ideally, every lesson should begin and end with success.

reinforcements for training

In order to make formal speech perception training palatable to the child, reinforcements are essential. After the child completes a set number of items, he can perform some agreeable activity. General rules for selecting reinforcements are listed below:

A. The child should be able to perform a reinforcement activity quickly; he should not spend more time with the reinforcement activity than with the training activity.

B. Reinforcement activities should not be too challenging or too absorbing; otherwise the child will not attend closely to the training task.

C. Activities must be varied; drawing lines on a paper may hold a child's interest for a few minutes, but the activity quickly wears thin.

D. Activities should interest the child; for example, if the child enjoys playing with money, he might drop coins into a bank.

E. The child should perform the reinforcement activity immediately after responding to a training item correctly.

F. Activities should be appropriate for the child's age and sex.

Verbal praise, a gentle touch, and smiling are wonderful reinforcers and should be used frequently. Training should be a positive experience. The teacher must never focus on *wrong* responses. Suggestions for training reinforcements appear in Table 5–2.

One teacher invented a *privilege book* to motivate her student. Each page in the privilege book contained fifteen squares. Every time the

Table 5–2:   Reinforcements That Can Be Used During Speech Perception Training.

Speech perception training reinforcements include:
- Drawing with chalk on a chalkboard,
- Dropping clothespins into a bottle,
- Collecting stickers,
- Spelling words with magnetic letters on a steel alphabet board,
- Playing with a *Mr. Potato Head*,
- Making animals or buildings with *Tinker Toys*, blocks, pipe cleaners, *Legos*, or *Duplos*,
- Building puzzles,
- Playing a card game,
- Dropping pennies into a bank,
- Placing pegs onto a pegboard,
- Arranging cutouts on a flannel board,
- Playing a board game,
- Coloring in a coloring book,
- Making popcorn or paper chains,
- Stringing beads into a necklace,
- Placing stars on a chart,
- Blowing soap bubbles,
- Playing musical instruments,
- Putting flowers into a vase,
- Earning tokens that can be used to purchase privileges, such as a trip to the library, five minutes of free time, an opportunity to write a letter,
- Earning tokens that can be used to purchase school supplies, such as pencils, notepads, and book covers.

---

child completed a set number of training items, the child placed a sticker on one of the squares. When a page was covered with squares, the child selected one of the privileges listed at the back of the book. Privileges included playing with clay, helping the teacher photocopy papers, pinning a drawing on the class bulletin board, engaging in five minutes of free time, operating the VHS machine, making a cover for a text book, choosing a book for the teacher to read, and taking a picture with a Polaroid camera. The teacher asked the child to review

Table 5-3: Suggestions for Speech Perception Training.

Suggestions for training include:
A. Repeat, repeat, repeat;

B. Provide many and varied speechreading and listening experiences;

C. Reinforce objectives from a formal lesson informally;

D. Respond to the child's vocalizations;

E. Have unlimited expectations;

F. Allow for spontaneity;

G. Often tell the child what you are going to say before he speechreads or listens;

H. Acknowledge the child's spontaneous responses to sound with praise and encouragement;

I. Stay alert to the child's focus of attention;

J. Do not introduce new vocabulary during speech perception training activities;

K. Set aside time every day for formal instruction;

L. Coordinate home and school efforts;

M. Capitalize on the child's interests and hobbies.

the list of privileges every time she made a new book, to ensure that he wanted to receive them.

guidelines for training

Table 5-3 presents a list of suggestions for conducting formal speech perception training.

The child must hear sounds many times before they become meaningful. He may recognize a sound one day but not the next. Sounds and speech materials should be presented in a variety of contexts, using many different activities.

The importance of responding to the child's vocalizations cannot be overstated. The child must become aware of his own voice, and realize that others respond to his vocalizations. These revelations are cornerstones for successful aural/oral communication. The child should be encouraged to vocalize as he signs.

Lesson plans may not always go according to plan, and the teacher must be flexible and allow for spontaneity. It is important that the teacher not limit the child's progress because of her limited expectations.

The teacher should frequently let the child know what she is going to say before she asks him to listen or to speechread. This will help him associate meaning with the auditory and audiovisual speech signals. For instance, the child can read a sentence before he speechreads it, or look at a corresponding picture illustration. He can speechread the teacher say a phrase or watch her speak and sign it before she covers her mouth during auditory training.

Spontaneous responses to sound should be met with praise and encouragement, particularly during the first months of implant use. During training, the teacher must be aware of the child's focus of attention and never attempt to incorporate vocabulary lessons with speech perception training activities.

Ten to thirty minutes should be set aside at the same time everyday for formal instruction; for example, before or after breakfast, before or after bathtime; before or after recess. This will make lessons part of the daily routine. Training should not be attempted when the child is tired. Parents should allow for "fun time," and not be overzealous in providing training.

Parents and teachers must coordinate their training efforts. They can maintain contact via occasional telephone calls and notes. One teacher developed a *Newsbook* for her student. In a small notebook, she wrote down what the child was doing in school. The child took the notebook home. The parents read the teacher's notes and then wrote about their training efforts. They also made comments about their son's home interests, hobbies, and any problems that he was having with his implant or communication skills. The notebook went back and forth between school and home about once a week.

Objectives from a formal lesson should be practiced informally throughout the day. For instance, one young implanted child discriminated a one-word utterance, *Hi!*, from a three-word utterance, *See you later!*,

Table 5–4: An Example of a Diary for Monitoring the Child's Interests.

Date: May 1
1. Interests
   A. Dinosaurs
   B. Cars
2. Hobbies
   A. Computers
   B. Jigsaw puzzles
3. Favorite toys and games
   A. Computer games
   B. Soccer
   C. Toy sports cars and motorcyles
4. Favorite television show and/or television characters
   A. Bronco Bill
   B. Batman Cartoons
5. Friends
   A. John Klein
   B. Theresa Adams
   C. Chris Jones
6. Activities that child is looking forward to
   A. Going to the roller skating rink in two weeks
   B. Summer camp
   C. John Klein's birthday party

during formal auditory training one morning with his mother. That night, his mother cheerfully said, "Hi!," as she appeared at his bedroom door. She said, "See you later!," as she stepped out of view. She repeated this several times, pausing long enough before reappearing so that the child responded to her voice rather than to her visual image. This activity reinforced the morning lesson, and was fun for both parent and child.

Training activities might be about a hobby or sport, such as soccer. This is a means for the parent or teacher to share the child's interests, and it also motivates the child during training. An interest diary like that presented in Table 5–4 can be used in designing training activities. The diary can be updated every few months.

summary

The goal of speech perception training is to develop the child's auditory and speechreading skills. Speech perception training can occur in individual or group sessions, and can be informal or formal. Informal training should initially occur during familiar routines, while talking about the here and now, and after establishing a context for aural/oral communication. In designing formal training activities, the parent or teacher must carefully select training materials, activities, and reinforcements.

references

Ling, D. (1988). *Foundations of Spoken Language for Hearing-Impaired Children*, Washington, D.C.: Alexander Graham Bell Association for the Deaf, Inc.
Tye-Murray, N., Tyler, R.S., Lansing, C., & Bertschy, M. (1990). Determining the effectiveness of auditory training stimuli using a computerized program. *Volta Review, 92,* 25–30.

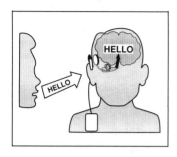

6

auditory training

nancy tye-murray, ph.d.
holly fryauf-bertschy, m.a.

The goal of auditory training is to develop the child's ability to hear and to understand speech. During training, the teacher does not encourage the child to monitor oral speech movements visually. In fact, the teacher may cover her mouth or speak from behind or beside the child.

This chapter first describes levels of auditory training tasks. It then presents guidelines for lesson objectives and training procedures. Finally, technology that can be used for training is briefly considered.

auditory training tasks

There are four levels of auditory training tasks: awareness, discrimination, identification, and comprehension (Erber, 1982).

awareness

The child with a new implant must first learn to detect the presence of sound. For a child who was born deaf or who lost his hearing early in life, it may take six months or more before he spontaneously responds to an auditory signal. Many parents and teachers feel discouraged and disappointed during this time. They must remember that the child must learn how to attend to sound.

The parent or teacher should make a point of showing her child the source and meaning of sounds, and reinforce the child when he responds to sound. Parents and teachers must become aware of sound themselves, and direct the child's attention toward it. They must learn to hear the world with new ears; for example, a parent might say:

"I here a loud noise. Look, its an airplane."

"I turned on the television. A woman is singing."

"I'm closing the refrigerator . . . listen. You try it."

"I hear Dad. He must be in the kitchen. Listen."

A child commonly increases his vocal play following implantation. For instance, he may frequently hum or produce repetitive syllables. Such vocalizations should not be discouraged. The child is becoming aware of his own voice, in much the fashion that an infant becomes aware of his voice through babbling.

discrimination

The second level of auditory training task requires the child to make gross sound discriminations. For instance, he might be asked to discriminate between *loud* and *soft* sounds, between *long* and *short* sounds, and between *high-pitched* and *low-pitched* sounds. He need not associate meaning with them.

Unless he progresses very slowly, the child should spend little time discriminating nonspeech sounds and nonsense syllables that differ suprasegmentally. Learning to distinguish between a high-pitched syllable sequence versus a low-pitched syllable sequence or a long tone versus a short tone may not build toward speech comprehension. Placing these discriminations in the context of meaningful speech units, as will be described later, is a more appropriate exercise.

identification

The third level of auditory training task requires finer discriminations and identification of speech stimuli. For instance, the child may be asked to label a word after hearing it, when provided with a set of four response choices.

comprehension

The final task in auditory training requires speech comprehension. The teacher might ask the child to answer questions or to follow directions. The child must identify what was said, interpret the meaning, and then respond appropriately.

Appendix 6–1 presents auditory training activities for each of the four levels. These activities are included in a handout that is provided to parents of implanted children at the University of Iowa Hospitals and Clinics.

environmental sounds and auditory training

During early implant use, nonspeech stimuli may be used to teach the child two important concepts. First, sound conveys meaning and second, action often produces sound. These concepts are best taught informally. For instance, a mother might give her son a set of pots and spoons. As the boy clangs the pots and silverware, he will hear his actions create sound. His mother can indicate when the sounds are soft and when they are loud. During an activity like this, the child should often control the sound source while the parent or teacher provides a commentary about the sounds. This will maintain his interest and lead to faster learning. Table 6–1 presents additional activities that present nonspeech stimuli.

speech and auditory training

A child who uses sign language has a visual representation of words. He must develop an auditory representation as well. When introducing a new vocabulary word, the teacher should teach its meaning and the articulatory gestures and speech sounds that are used to produce it. The child's developing awareness of the spoken and oral representations of words may be closely related to his ability to identify them auditorily.

Once the child begins to respond to sound consistently, auditory training should be directed toward developing speech discrimination, identifi-

Table 6–1:   Objects That Can Be Used to Teach the Child That Sound Has Meaning and That Action Often Produces Sound.

- Blender filled with water and ice cubes
- Hammer and peg toy
- Set of keys
- Whistle
- Drum and drumsticks
- Bell
- Toilet flushing
- Water faucet
- Pots and pans
- Hair dryer
- Vacuum cleaner
- Piano
- Harmonica
- Tambourine
- Doorbell
- Hand clapping
- Music box

cation, and comprehension. Lessons can include one of two kinds of activities, or both. One kind requires the child to attend to phonetic-level information and the other requires him to attend to word- and sentence-level information (Stout & Windle, 1986).

The rate at which the objectives are achieved will vary greatly from child to child. Often, progress will be slow and will occur in a dramatic "spurt" when it is least expected. Progress will be influenced by the child's age at implantation, the amount of hearing experience he had prior to receiving an implant, his auditory capabilities with the device, the consistency of the parents and teachers over time in providing auditory stimulation, and whether or not the training tasks are enjoyable for the child.

phonetic-level auditory training objectives

There are two kinds of phonetic-level auditory training objectives, vowel and consonant. In this section, we will consider the acoustic properties of vowels and consonants, and present specific training objectives and materials.

vowel auditory training objectives

Vowel Formants: The vowel auditory training objectives are designed to contrast vowels with different formants. Vowel formants are the result of vocal tract resonances that cause more energy to be produced at some frequencies than others. Each vowel has at least two characteristic formants, the first and second formant. It is the combination of these formants that causes one vowel to sound different from another.

The first formant is determined by how opened is the mouth. For instance, a relatively opened mouth shape, such as that for /a/ (as in *odd*), usually results in a first formant with high frequency. More closed mouth openings, such as those associated with /i/ (as in *heed*) and /u/ (as in *who*), result in low-frequency first formants.

The frequency of the second formant is determined greatly by whether the tongue is placed more forward or more backward in the mouth. Forward tongue displacement produces a high frequency second formant; for example, /i/. Tongue displacement toward the back of the mouth produces a low-frequency second formant; for example, /u/. Typical first and second formant values for the vowels of English are listed in Table 6–2.

The Cochlear Corporation Nucleus cochlear implant is specifically designed to code the vowel formants. The speech processor receives the speech signal from the microphone and then identifies the frequency values of the first and second formants. The new version of the Nucleus processor, called the MSP strategy, also codes a third vowel formant. The frequencies of the formants of voiced sounds determine which of the device's twenty-two electrodes will be stimulated.

Early auditory training should focus the child's attention on discriminating vowels since this information is readily available to the implant user. Moreover, research has shown that if a cochlear implant user can identify vowels fairly well, he will likely be able to identify sentences relatively well (Tyler, Tye-Murray, & Gantz, 1987).

Vowel Awareness: Initial vowel auditory training should be directed toward developing the child's awareness of different vowel sounds. Young children can use toys such as a cow and lamb (Ling, 1976), and

Table 6–2: Typical Frequency Values of the First and Second Vowel Formants, Spoken by an Adult Male Talker (from Peterson & Barney, 1952).

Vowel	Example	First Formant (Hz)	Second Formant (Hz)
/i/	beet	270	2290
/I/	bit	390	1990
/ɛ/	bet	530	1840
/æ/	bat	660	1720
/a/	box	730	1090
/ɔ/	ball	570	840
/U/	book	440	1020
/u/	boot	300	870
/ʌ/	but	640	1190
/3ⁿ/	bird	490	1350

listen as the cow makes a *mooo* sound and the lamb makes a *baaah* sound. A train will make a *choo choo* sound and a tugboat will make a *chug chug* sound.

The child and teacher can take turns babbling consecutive syllable strings with different vowels, one string right after the other; for example, *ba ba ba, bee bee bee, boo boo boo*. The teacher can vocalize one vowel and then smoothly change to another vowel; for example, *eeeeeuuuuu*. The child's task is to indicate when the vowel changes by pointing to one of two colors, each corresponding to one of the two vowels. The child should also vocalize the vowel pair. These procedures should be repeated with a variety of pairs.

Vowel Discrimination and Identification: After the child demonstrates vowel awareness, training objectives can require him to discriminate and identify vowel stimuli. The vowel training objectives presented below are similar to those described in the *Developmental Approach to Successful Listening* (DASL) (Stout & Windle, 1986) auditory training program:

1. The child will discriminate vowels that differ in first formant information, using a two-item response set; for example, *beet* from *bat*.

Table 6–3: Vowel and Word Pairs That Can Be Used for Achieving the First Vowel Auditory Training Objective: *The Child Will Discriminate Vowels That Differ in First Formant Information.*

A. Vowel pairs[1]

/u/ (*boot*) versus /ɛ/ (*bet*), /æ/ (*bat*), /ʌ/ (*but*), or /a/ (*box*)

/U/ (*hood*) versus /ɛ/, /æ/, /ʌ/, or /a/

/i/ (*bead*) versus /ɛ/, /æ/, /ʌ/, or /a/

/I/ (pin) versus /ɛ/, /æ/, /ʌ/, or /a/

B. Word pairs

shoe/shop	tune/ten	pin/pig
bee/bat	tooth/tap	moon/men
boot/bat	shoe/shut	put/pet
book/back	put/pot	bead/bed
pin/pen	seed/sad	feet/fat
rib/rub	big/bug	shoe/shop
dream/drum	spill/spell	hit/hat

---

2. The child will discriminate vowels that differ in second formant information, using a two-item response set; for example, *beet* from *boot*.

3. The child will discriminate words that have vowels with similar first and second formant information, using a two-item response set; for example, *mail* from *mill*.

4. The child will identify words with different vowels, using a four-item response set; for example, *beet* from the response set of: *beet*, *boot*, *bat*, and *bet*.

5. The child will identify words with different vowels, from an open set of familiar vocabulary.

Objectives 1–3: Tables 6–3, 6–4, and 6–5 present vowel and word pairs that can be used for achieving the first three objectives. In a typical discrimination activity, the child has before him two pictures; for example, one of a beet and one of a bat. He might place a penny on the appropriate picture every time the teacher says one of the two words. The child must respond correctly 35 of 40 times before moving on to the next pair. When

---

[1]For the first occurrence of each target sound in this and the following tables, an example of a word containing the sound is presented

Table 6–4: Vowel and Word Pairs That Can Be Used For Achieving The Second Vowel Auditory Training Objective: *The Child Will Discriminate Vowels That Differ in Second Formant Information.*

A. Vowel pairs

/i/ (*bee*) versus /u/ (*boo*)

/o/ (*pole*) versus /e/ (*pale*) or /$3^\cap$/ (*pearl*)

/e/ versus /$3^\cap$/

/ɔ/ (*lawn*) versus /e/ or /$3^\cap$/

/a/ (*pod*) versus /æ/ (*pad*)

/U/ (*pull*) versus /I/ (*pill*)

B. Word pairs

bee/boo	low/lay	low/learn
fawn/fern	hot/hat	book/bit
me/moo	shock/shake	lock/lake
row/ray	mean/moon	feel/fool
he/who	saw/sat	coat/cake
look/lick	dawn/dirt	knee/new
beet/boot	pot/pat	pull/pill

possible, five word pairs should be used with a vowel pair. For instance, *beet* and *boot*, *leap* and *loop*, *see* and *Sue*, *tea* and *two*, and *knee* and *new* can be used for contrasting /i/ and /u/. All vowel pairs listed in the tables should be practiced for each objective.

If the child has difficulty in discriminating a stimuli pair, he can first practice speechreading the items with a *same/different* task. Figure 6–1 presents a response illustration that a teacher can photocopy. It has a picture indicating *same* and one indicating *different*. The teacher can speak two words or phrases, such as *That's a pop/That's a peep* or *That's a pop/That's a pop*. The child then indicates whether the stimuli are the same or different by touching the appropriate picture or by placing a penny on it.

Ideally, the words used in a discrimination task should be alike except for the contrasting sounds; for example, the child might discriminate *beet* from *bat*, where the two vowels are contrasting. Such word pairs

Table 6–5:   Vowel and Word Pairs That Can Be Used for Achieving the Third Vowel Auditory Training Objective: *The Child Will Discriminate Vowels With Similar First and Second Formant Information.*

A. Vowel pairs

/o/ (*woke*) versus /ɔ/ (*walk*)

/I/ (*sit*) versus /i/ (*seat*)

/e/ (*shape*) versus /I/ (*ship*)

/ɛ/ (*met*) versus /e/ (*mate*)

/a/ (*cop*) versus /ʌ/ (*cup*)

B. Word pairs

pen/pain	hot/hut	lawn/lone
shape/ship	mit/meat	phone/fawn
fed/fade	net/knit	shed/shade
fit/feet	get/gate	bowl/ball
tin/teen	pet/paid	hog/hug
wet/wait	ship/sheep	show/shawl
mitt/meat	chip/cheap	rod/rug

---

are relatively easy to construct when the child can read and has an extensive vocabulary. However, when the child cannot read, pictures or objects must be available so that he can respond by touching a representation of the word. It is often difficult to identify simple word pairs that can be illustrated. Occasionally, the words will have to be similar, but contrast by more than one sound; for example, *book* versus *beet*, where the contrasting vowels are /U/ and /i/. Table 6–6 presents a list of common one-syllable words that can be illustrated and used for vowel auditory training.

Objectives 4 and 5: For the fourth objective, the response sets increase from two to four choices; for example, the teacher might say the word *beet*. The child's task is to touch one of four pictures: a beet, a boot, a bat, or a bed. Toys or objects may be used in place of pictures.

A means of introducing stimuli for a closed-set identification activity, as required in Objective 4, is by using a *Concentration* game format with flashcards. The flashcards can represent the words that will be practiced

Table 6–6:   Words That Can Be Illustrated and Used For Vowel Auditory Training Exercises.

/u/		/U/		/i/	
soup	goose	book	hood	beak	geese
boot	tool	hook	wood	wheat	feet
food	moon	foot	pull	beat	peel
suit	pool	full	shook	seat	sheet
shoe	fool	bull	cook	bean	meat
/I/		**/ɛ/**		**/æ/**	
bit	men	net	head	bat	fat
sit	mitt	bell	men	bag	gas
lid	pill	wet	red	man	hat
pin	kick	bed	pet	mat	pan
/ʌ/		**/a/**		**/3ⁿ/**	
gun	up	shot	doll	bird	turn
pup	one	top	sock	shirt	girl
cut	bun	rock	knot	burn	curve
run	gun	hot	hop	pearl	purse
/e/		**/o/**		**/ɔ/**	
rake	cake	bow	coat	shawl	lawn
eight	rain	note	bone	long	fawn
lake	cave	pole	boat	dawn	ball
tape	bait	hose	goat	walk	chalk

in the identification activity. The flashcards should be placed face down on a table. Every time the child touches one, the teacher turns it over and says the name of the picture. The child should repeat the word after the teacher. This process continues until all cards have been turned face-up. Once the child is familiar with the set of words, he can be asked to identify them in a closed-set identification format.

For the fifth objective, the child must identify words using an open-set format; that is, without a set of response choices. In one exercise, the child might identify words whose vowels have a high-frequency second formant; for example, *bat*, *bet*, *bait*, *bit*, and *beet*. The teacher might say, "That's a bat," and ask the child to repeat the word without having before him a group of words or pictures from which to choose.

consonant auditory training objectives

Consonant Features: The consonant auditory training objectives are based on contrasting three features of articulation: manner, place of production, and voicing. *Manner* is used to classify consonants by the kind of articulatory movements that are used to produce them. For instance, some consonants are produced with slow movements (the glides), such as the /l/ in *land*. Some are produced by forcing air through a small opening (the fricatives), such as the /f/ in *fan*. *Place* refers to where in the mouth the primary constriction occurs. Traditional place classifications are bilabial, such as the /b/ in *ban* (the two lips meet during sound production), labiodental, such as /f/ (the lower lip contacts the upper teeth), linguadental, such as the /θ/ in *thumb* (the tongue tip contacts the upper teeth), alveolar, such as the /t/ in *tan* (the tongue tip approximates or touches the roof of the mouth, just behind the teeth), palatal such as the /ʃ/ in *sheep* (the midsection of the tongue approximates or touches the roof of the mouth), and velar, such as the /k/ in *key* (the back of the tongue approximates or touches the roof of the mouth). *Voicing* indicates whether or not the vocal cords vibrate during the consonant constriction.

Table 6–7 presents a list of constants grouped together according to place of production, manner, and voice. Traditional groupings have been modified in order to simplify speech perception training. For place of production, consonants that are traditionally considered palatal (/ʃ, j, dʒ, tʃ/) have been grouped together with velar consonants (/k, g/). Fricatives (/f, θ, s, ʃ, h, v, ð, z/) and affricatives have been grouped together (/tʃ, dʒ/).

Consonants can be classified into five different manner groups: stops, nasals, fricatives, glides, and affricatives. Stop consonants such as /p, b/ are produced with complete closure of the mouth, allowing pressure to build up behind the constriction. They are often released with a quick burst of air. Stops are relatively soft or low-amplitude segments of speech. They can be produced with or without voicing.

Nasal consonants such as /n, m/ are produced by lowering the velum and allowing air to flow through the nose. Nasal consonants have a low-frequency resonance, which is referred to as a nasal murmur. Most implant users can detect this information. Nasals are louder than stops or fricatives, and are always produced with voice.

Table 6–7: Consonants Grouped By Place of Production, Manner, and Voice.

A. Consonants differing in manner
   Stops: /p, b, t, d, k, g/
   Fricatives and affricatives: /f, v, θ, ð , h, s, ʃ, z, dʒ, tʃ/
   Nasals: /m, n/
   Liquids and glides: /w, j, r, l/

B. Consonants differing in voicing
   Voiced: /b, d, g, dʒ, v, ð , z, m, n, l, w, j, r/
   Unvoiced: /p, t, k, tʃ, f, θ, h, s, ʃ/

C. Consonants differing in place of production
   Bilabial: /m, p, b, w/
   Labiodental: /f, v/
   Linguadental: / ð , θ/
   Alveolar: /t, d, s, z, n, l/
   Velar and palatal: /k, g, ʃ, j, dʒ, tʃ, h/

Fricatives such as /s, z/ are produced by forcing the breath stream through a small opening in the mouth, thereby creating a turbulent airflow. Fricatives often have a hissing sound. Fricatives are longer in duration and louder than stops. They can be produced with or without voice. An affricative is produced by combining a stop with a fricative.

The glides are produced with slow articulatory gestures. The sounds /w, j, r/ require a small mouth opening whereas /l/ requires a more open mouth opening. The glides are louder than stops and fricatives and are always voiced.

Adult cochlear implant users can often hear voicing and nasality cues. For instance, they will likely be able to distinguish *tip* from *dip*, and *mat* from *bat*. Less often, they can determine whether or not a consonant is a fricative. For instance, they may or may not be able to distinguish *fit* from *pit*. The most difficult speech cues to discriminate are those that pertain to place of production. A cochlear implant user often has great difficulty distinuishing *bun* from *done* from *gun*. These three words are all voiced stops, and differ only in place of production within the mouth.

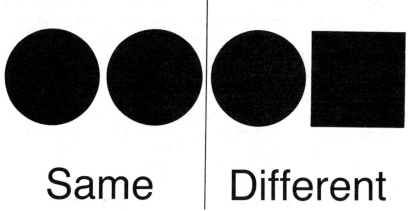

Same | Different

Figure 6–1: **A response illustration for a same/different task that can be photocopied and used for auditory training.**

Consonant Awareness: Initial training should develop the child's awareness of consonant sounds. The child must recognize that the speech signal contains loud segments (vowels) and soft segments (consonants). Training can begin with activities similar to those proposed for developing vowel awareness.

Voiceless fricatives have a relatively long duration. They contrast with voiced vowel segments because they have low amplitude. The teacher can vocalize a vowel, inserting a voiceless fricative (/s, ʃ, f/) in the middle; for example, *eeeeesheeeee*. The child can then imitate her production. He can do this with a variety of vowels.

Next, the teacher can present a prolonged vowel and a vowel interpreted by a voiceless fricative. The child's task to indicate whether the two stimuli are the *same* or *different* using the response illustration shown in Figure 6–1. For instance, the teacher might say, "Eeeeeeeeeee", and then, "Eeeefeeee." In this example, the child should touch the *different* illustration. The talker should produce items in a same/different task with equal duration, loudness, and pitch.

After the child has performed these tasks consistently wth voiceless fricatives, he may repeat them with voiceless stops (/p, t, k/), nasals (/m, n/), and then voiced fricatives (/z, v/). These sounds are increasingly difficult to distinguish from the flanking vowel context, either because they have shorter duration or greater amplitude than voiceless fricatives.

The teacher and the child can take turns babbling syllable strings with different initial consonants; for example, *sa sa sa*, *ma ma ma*, *la la la*. Different vowel contexts should be used; for example, *see see see*. The child should hear the strings first while seeing the teacher's face and then repeat them. He should then listen without seeing her face.

Discrimination and Identification Objectives: After awareness training, training exercises should include consonant ensembles that differ in manner and voice and/or place of production, for instance, /t, m, g/; /s, n, b/, because these sounds differ greatly from one another acoustically. Consonants that differ in place of production but share manner and voice, for instance, /b, d, g/, should be included fairly late since they are difficult to distinguish using only the auditory signal.

The objectives for consonant discrimination and identification activities progress in the following order:

1. The child will discriminate nasal versus non-nasal unvoiced consonants that differ in place of production; for example, *meat* from *seat*.
2. The child will discriminate nasal versus non-nasal voiced consonants that differ in place of production; for example, *map* from *gap*.
3. The child will discriminate unvoiced fricatives versus voiced stops that differ in place of production; for example, *son* from *gun*.
4. The child will discriminate unvoiced fricatives versus unvoiced stops that differ in place of production; *sea* from *key*.
5. The child will identify words whose consonants share manner of production from a four-item and then six-item response set; for example, *sat* from the response set of: *sat*, *fat*, *shot*, and *van*.
6. The child will identify words whose consonants are all either voiced or unvoiced from a four-item and then six-item response set; for example, *cat* from the response set of: *cat*, *pat*, *tap*, and *sack*.
7. The child will identify words whose consonants share place of production from a four-item and then six-item response set; for example, *pat* from the response set of: *pat*, *mat*, *bat*, and *fat*.
8. The child will identify words in an open-set of familiar vocabulary words.

Tables 6–8, 6–9, 6–10, and 6–11 present consonant and word pairs that can be used for achieving the first four objectives. When possible,

Table 6–8: Consonant and Word Pairs That Can Be Used for Achieving the First Consonant Auditory Training Objective: *The Child Will Discriminate Nasal Versus Non-Nasal Unvoiced Consonants That Differ in Place of Production.*

A. Consonant pairs

/m/ (*me*) versus /ʃ/ (*she*), /s/ (*sea*), /t/ (*tea*), /k/ (*key*),
/tʃ/ (*cheese*), /h/ (*he*), /f/ (*fee*)
/n/ (*knee*) versus /p/ (*pea*), /k/, /f/, /h/, /ʃ/

B. Word pairs

meat/seat	malt/salt	near/fear
net/pet	milk/silk	note/coat
mail/tail	money/sunny	news/shoes
noon/coon	nap/tap	might/sight
new/shoe	nose/toes	might/fight
man/fan	neat/feet	no/so
may/say	mat/sat	no/toe

Table 6–9: Consonant and Word Pairs That Can Be Used for Achieving the Second Consonant Auditory Training Objective: *The Child Will Discriminate Nasal Versus Non-Nasal Voiced Consonants That Differ in Place of Production.*

A. Consonant pairs

/m/ (*me*) versus /d/ (*D*), /g/ (*geese*), /dʒ/ (*jeep*),
/l/ (*leap*), /w/ (*weep*), /r/ (*reap*)
/n/ (*knee*) versus /b/ (*bee*), /g/, /w/, /r/

B. Word pairs

nail/rail	near/gear	near/dear
moose/goose	mice/dice	kneel/deal
nap/lap	mow/dough	nail/bail
nine/wine	net/jet	make/lake
mall/doll	nice/dice	knot/dot
note/goat	net/debt	knit/bit
mail/whale	neigh/day	make/rake

Table 6–10:   Consonant and Word Pairs That Can Be Used for Achieving the Third Consonant Auditory Training Objective: *The Child Will Discriminate Unvoiced Fricatives Versus Voiced Stops That Differ in Place of Production.*

A. Consonant pairs
/f/ (*fate*) versus /d/ (*date*), /g/ (*gate*)
/s/ (*sun*) versus /b/ (*bun*), /g/
/h/ (*he*) versus /b/, /d/
/ʃ/ (*she*) versus /b/, /d/

B. Word pairs

fun/gun	sell/bell	same/game
shoe/dew	heart/dart	fog/dog
hit/bit	sack/back	shoot/boot
hat/bat	song/gone	shed/bed
sun/gun	fall/doll	hay/day
fat/gas	shake/bake	fish/dish
shine/dime	she/bee	head/bed

five different sets of stimuli should be presented for each consonant pair in a discrimination task. The child's vocabulary may limit the number of stimuli pairs that can be used for training. The child should respond correctly to thirty five of forty presentations before proceeding to the next pair. Table 6–12 presents a list of common one-syllable words that can be illustrated, which can be used for consonant auditory training. These words can be used with children who cannot read.

After the objectives have been achieved with consonants in the initial position, exercises can include them in the final position of words. A carrier phrase such as, *That's a ___.*, can be used for presenting noun stimuli.

word- and sentence-level auditory training objectives

Comprehension of sentences and connected discourse using only the auditory signal will be the most difficult task the child will be asked to achieve. The process of teaching the child to recognize sentences

Table 6–11: Consonant and Word Pairs That Can Be Used for Achieving the Fourth Consonant Auditory Training Objective: *The Child Will Discriminate Unvoiced Fricatives Versus Unvoiced Stops That Differ in Place of Production.*

A. Consonant pairs

/f/ (as in *fee*) versus /t/ (*tea*), /k/ (*key*)

/s/ (*sat*) versus /p/ (*pat*), /k/

/h/ (*hop*) versus /p/, /t/

/ʃ/ (*shop*) versus /p/, /t/

B. Word pairs

fall/tall	hat/pat	fin/tin
seal/peel	shine/pine	soil/coil
hat/pat	face/cake	hay/pay
ship/pick	phone/cone	show/toe
shell/tell	sing/king	same/came
fan/tan	heart/part	she/tea
sand/can	shake/take	fat/cat

auditorily can start by asking him to discriminate short utterances from long utterances; for example, *a cat* versus *a big brown dog.*

Then exercises can included activities where two pictures are set before the child. The teacher can speak a sentence that describes one; for example, *The cat is on the fence.* The child's task is to select the correct picture after hearing the sentence. Initially she can say it with her face visible and then without her face visible. As the child progresses, more pictures can be included as possible responses, and the descriptions can be presented auditorily first.

Next the child can follow simple directions, first with a closed set of responses and then with an open set (Stout & Windle, 1985). For instance, the child might be asked to color a box *red* when he has before him a red and yellow crayon. Later, he may have before him the entire box of crayons. The child can be asked to point to body parts following auditory instructions; for example, *Show me your nose., Show me your elbow., Show me your ear.*

Once he can perform these activities, he can answer simple questions; for example, *How are you?, How old are you?, What's your name?.*

Table 6–12: Words That Can Be Illustrated and Used For Consonant Auditory Training Exercises.

/p/		/b/		/t/	
pan	pea	bee	boot	tea	tool
peach	pick	ball	bell	top	team
pool	pill	bat	boat	tooth	top
pop	pin	beet	bed	tack	toad

/d/		/k/		/g/	
dog	clock	K	can	gas	gum
dad	dough	cop	cap	goose	game
dot	ditch	cook	keys	geese	girl
doll	D	cat	cob	gun	goat

/tʃ/		/dʒ/		/f/	
church	cheer	jar	J	fat	fall
chair	chew	jump	jack	foot	feet
chick	chain	jeep	jeans	fan	fox
chin	cheek	jet	juice	fish	face

/v/		/θ/			
vase	vault	thumb	three		
van	vane	thigh	thick		
veil	vest	thin	thorn		
vine	valve	thread	thief		

/h/		/s/		/ʃ/	
hot	hay	seat	sail	sheep	shorts
hit	house	suit	sock	shoes	shirt
ham	hip	sack	sew	sheet	shack
heel	hand	seed	soup	shell	ship

		/m/		/n/	
		mouse	moon	nail	net
		men	mat	knot	nap
		man	mice	knees	neck
		mail	match	kneel	nose

/l/		/w/		/r/	
leg	lamp	wet	web	red	rice
loop	leaf	wig	witch	rain	rose
lamb	light	wave	wire	rake	wrap
lock	lime	wine	wood	run	rock

An appropriate context should be established before the questions are presented auditorily. If the child learns to recognize picture descriptions and directions auditorily, lesson objectives can finally focus on teaching him to comprehend narratives.

The objectives for word- and sentence-level auditory training are listed below. Many children will not achieve all of the objectives. Some may only achieve a few.

1. The child will discriminate multiword utterances from single-word utterances, using a closed response set; for example, *How are you today?* from *Hi!*. Later, he can be asked to discriminate long words from short words; for example, *Halloween* from *cat*.

2. The child will discriminate a spondee from a one-syllable word; for example, *ice cream* from *shoe*. Later, he can be asked to discriminate a spondee from a two-syllable word; for example, *toothbrush* from *pony*.

3. The child will discriminate between words having the same number of syllables; for example, *cat* from *dog*.

4. The child will identify simple words from a four-item and then a six-item response set; for example, *cat* from the response set of *cat*, *dog*, *elephant*, and *camel*.

5. The child will identify picture illustrations from a closed-set, after hearing one-sentence descriptions.

6. The child will follow simple directions and answer simple questions, using a closed response set.

7. The child will listen to two related sentences, and then draw a picture about them; for example, he might draw a picture after hearing, *The boy is playing. He has a ball.*

A list of long and short stimuli pair is presented in Table 6–13. The pairs can be used for achieving Objective 1. A list of spondee words appears in Table 6–14. The spondees can be used for achieving Objective 2.

conducting a formal lesson

The objectives are designed to be completed in order, but the teacher can change the order if it seems warranted by the child's performance.

Table 6–13:   Long and Short Stimuli Pairs That Can Be Used for Achieving the First Objective of Word- and Sentence-Level Auditory Training: *The Child Will Discriminate Multiword Utterances from Single-Word Utterances; Long Words From Short Words.*

- What is your name/hi
- Brush your teeth/smile
- How are you/bye
- Beat the drum/whistle
- Give me a puzzle piece/draw
- A big brown bear/a cat
- A box of crayons/a can
- A glass of water/salt
- A yellow sweater/sock
- Table and chairs/stool
- Jack-O-Lantern/cat
- Santa Claus/tree
- Bicycle/skate
- Applesauce/grape
- Motorcycle/car

The training materials need not be elaborate or require a great deal of preparation time. Some teachers keep a three-ring notebook with pictures arranged in alphabetical order; for example, a picture of a baseball, a boy, a cat, and so forth. Whenever they find a colorful, uncluttered picture, they tear it from the magazine and glue it to a piece of notebook paper. These pictures are then readily available for training activities.

Lessons should occur in a quiet place with minimal distractions. If the child is seated at a table, it should be cleared of everything but the training materials and reinforcers. Siblings, friends, or classmates should not be present unless they are part of the lesson plan.

The teacher should not obscure her mouth by covering it with her hand or heavy paper since this will attenuate her speech (Niday & Elfenbein, 1991). If she is sitting across from the child, she can hide her mouth with a mesh screen or dark netting placed between embroidery hoops (Figure 6–2, p. 112). The teacher should try to stay within four to twelve inches

Table 6–14: Two-Syllable Words That Can Be Used for Achieving the Second Objective of Word- and Sentence-Level Auditory Training: *The Child Will Discriminate a Two-Syllable from a One-Syllable Word; from a Two Part Word.*

airplane	lamp post	Star Wars
bandaid	light bulb	sunshine
baseball	maltball	thumbtack
Batman	milkshake	toothbrush
blackboard	mousetrap	
boxcar	pancake	
cowboy	popcorn	
cupcake	railroad	
fence post	raindrop	
fisherman	runway	
flashlight	sailboat	
football	sandwich	
french fry	schoolhouse	
grandson	shoebox	
greenhouse	shoestring	
greyhound	sidewalk	
gumstick	snowball	
hotdog	snowcone	
horseshoe	snowman	
houseboat	spaceship	
ice cream	stairwell	

of the child's microphone. A good location is next to the child, on the side that he wears the microphone.

audio tape-card machines and tape recorders

Auditory training lessons may include audiotaped materials, using either a tape recorder or an audio tape-card machine (Erber, 1976; Sims, 1978). An attractive feature of audio tape-card machines (Figure 6–3) is that familiar vocabulary and familiar voices, such as a sibling's or parent's, may be recorded on tape cards and used for training. In this manner, the child learns to recognize the speech of those he interacts with most fre-

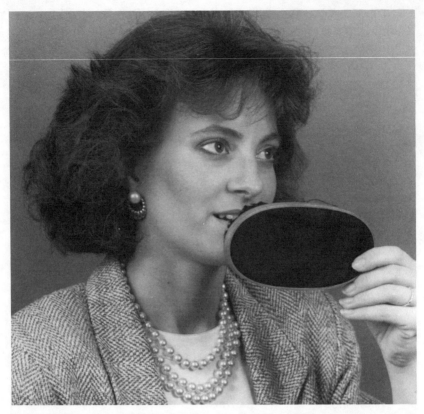

**Figure 6–2: A teacher obscuring her visible speech movements
with a meshscreen.**

quently. In addition, by using a tape-card machine, the child can hear
several different talkers during the same lesson.

Some implanted children enjoy having their own tape recorders. They can
manipulate the control panels, and choose which tapes to play. Several
inexpensive, child-proof models are available commercially. The child can
listern to tapes of nursery rhymes and songs. Musical arrangements should
be simple, with few instruments and little or no choral singing. The child
can be encouraged to sway in rhythm with music and even to sing along.
If the child has a postlingual hearing loss, he can listen to familiar songs
that he enjoyed prior to losing his hearing; for example, *The Happy Birthday Song* or *Twinkle Twinkle Little Star* (adult implant users report that
they enjoy listening to familiar songs more than unfamiliar songs). Re-

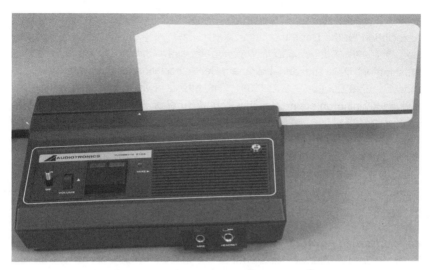

Figure 6–3:   An audiotape-card machine.

corded stories with accompanying books are enjoyable for some children, especially when the books are well-illustrated and have simple vocabulary.

summary

There are four levels of auditory training tasks: awareness, discrimination, identification, and comprehension. Whenever possible, the tasks should be performed with meaningful speech stimuli.

An auditory training exercise can include phonetic-level and word- and sentence-level objectives. Phonetic-level objectives should first require the child to attend to speech contrasts that are relatively easy to detect; for example, consonant voicing. They should ultimately require him to attend to information that is relatively difficult to detect; for example, consonant place of production. Word-level objectives should progress from presenting simple words and phrases to presenting sentences and short narratives auditorily.

references

Erber, N. (1976). The use of audio tapecards in auditory training for hearing-impaired children. *The Volta Review, 78*, 209–218.

Erber, N. (1982). *Auditory Training*. Washington, D. C.: Alexander Graham Bell Association for the Deaf, Inc.

Ling, D. (1976). *Speech and the Hearing-impaired Child: Theory and Practice*. Washington, D.C.: Alexander Graham Bell Association for the Deaf, Inc.

Niday, K. J., & Elfenbein, J. L. (1991). The effects of visual barriers used during auditory training on sound transmission. *Journal of Speech and Hearing Research, 34.* 694–696.

Peterson, G., & Barney, H. (1952). Control methods used in a study of vowels. *Journal of the Acoustical Society of America, 24*, 175–184.

Sims, D. G. (1978). Visual and auditory training for adults. In J. Katz (Ed.), *Handbook of Clinical Audiology (Second edition),* Baltimore: Williams & Wilkins.

Stout, G. G., & Windle, J. V. E. (1986). *The Developmental Approach to Successful Listening (DASL).* Houston: Stout & Windle.

Tyler, R. S., Tye-Murray, N., & Grantz, B. J. (1988). The relationship between vowel, consonant, and word perception in cochlear-implant patients. *Proceedings of the International Cochlear Implant Symposium, Duren, West Germany, 1987,* P. Banfai (Ed.), West Germany: Fachbuchhandlung, 627–632.

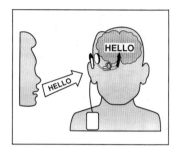

7

speechreading training
nancy tye-murray, ph.d.

Few individuals who hear normally appreciate how difficult it is to recognize speech visually. Only about 40 percent of speech sounds are clearly visible on the face. A talker produces approximately thirteen to fifteen articulatory gestures per second yet the eye can only register about eight or nine. Many words look alike and their appearance may change with sentence context and different talkers.

Despite these limitations, the visual signal significantly helps cochlear implant recipients understand speech. They can understand more when they speechread (use both the auditory and visual signals) than when they listen (use only the auditory signal). Figure 7–1 presents results from a sentence test that was completed by sixteen adults who use the Nucleus cochlear implant. On average, the implanted adults recognized 39 percent of the words using only audition. When they heard and viewed the talker at the same time (the audition-plus-vision condition), they recognized 83 percent of the words.

The purpose of speechreading training is to develop a child's ability to recognize speech audiovisually. During the first year or two of

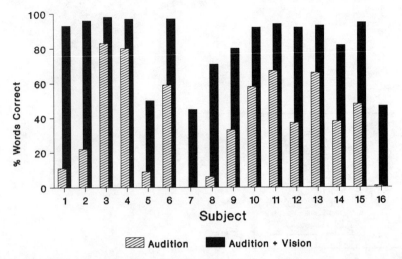

Figure 7–1: **Results from the Iowa Laser Videodisc Sentence Test (Tyler, Preece, & Tye-Murray, 1986), which contains one hundred sentences. The subjects heard a sentence and then attempted to repeat it verbatim. The number of words correctly repeated was tallied for a percentage score for each subject.**

implant use, a formal speechreading lesson should include both phonetic-level and sentence-level objectives. As the child's skills develop, lessons can present only sentence materials. This chapter describes phonetic-level and sentence-level objectives and then briefly considers technology that can be used in training.

phonetic-level speechreading training objectives

As with auditory training, there are two types of speechreading training objectives, vowel and consonant. In this section, the visual properties of speech sounds are considered, and specific vowel and consonant training objectives and materials are presented.

visemes

Sounds that look alike on the face are called *visemes*; for example, /p/ (as in *pat*), /b/ (*bat*), and /m/ (*mat*). Consonant and vowel viseme groups are presented in Table 7–1. One goal of speechreading train-

Table 7–1: Viseme Groups.

A. Consonant viseme groups

/p, b, m/

/f, v/

/ ð, θ/

/ʃ, ʒ, tʃ, dʒ/

/t, d, s, z, j, k, n, g, l/

B. Vowel and diphthong viseme groups

/u, U, o/

/aU/

/ɔ, ɔl/

/i, I, e, ∧, ε, æ, a, al/

---

ing is to teach the child to use the auditory signal to distinguish members in the same viseme category.

Consonants can be classified into at least six different viseme categories (Walden, Erdman, Montgomery, Schwartz, & Prosek, 1981). The phonemes /p, b, m/ are produced with the lips pressed together. The lower lip contacts the upper teeth when producing /f/ (*face*) and /v/ (*vase*). The phonemes /θ/ (*thick*) and / ð / (*thee*) are produced with the tongue tip pressed against the upper teeth, and /ʃ/ (*she*), /ʒ/ (*azure*), /tʃ/ (*cheese*), and /dʒ/ (*jeep*) are produced with the lips rounded and slightly protruded. The phonemes /w/ (*weed*) and /r/ (*reed*) require the talker to pucker the lips into a narrow opening. The movements of several consonants are obscure or invisible: /t/ (*tea*), /d/ (*deep*), /s/ (*sea*), /z/ (*zeal*), /j/ (*yeast*), /k/ (*key*), /n/ (*knee*), /g/ (*geese*), and /l/ (*leap*).

Vowels and diphthongs (such as the /aU/ sound in *how*) can be classified into at least four viseme categories (Jeffers & Barley, 1971). The lips pucker and form a narrow opening for /u/ (*who*), /U/ (*hook*), and /o/ (*hoe*). They relax and form a moderate opening, and then pucker to form a narrow opening for /aU/ (*how*). For the sounds /ɔ/ (*dawn*) and /ɔl/ (*boy*), the lips round with a moderate opening. The lips relax and form a narrow opening for /i/ (*heed*), /ɪ/ (*hid*), /e/ (*hay*), /ʌ/ (*hud*), /ɛ/ (*head*), /æ/ (*had*), /a/ (*hot*), and /aɪ/ (*high*).

vowel speechreading training objectives

As Chapter 6 explained, resonances in the mouth result in some frequencies (or pitches) having more energy than other frequencies. All vowels have characteristic high-energy frequency bands called *formants*. The frequency of the first and second formants greatly determine how a vowel sounds.

Vowel-level speechreading training should begin by teaching the child to distinguish /i/ (as in *heed*), /u/ (*who*), and /a/ (*odd*). These sounds differ visually and acoustically. The /i/ sound is produced with relaxed lips and a narrow mouth opening. It has a low-frequency first formant and a high-frequency second formant. The sound /u/ is produced with lips puckered and a narrow opening, and has a low-frequency first and second formant. A moderate opening and relaxed lips are associated with /a/. This vowel has mid-range frequency values for both first and second formants.

The vowel speechreading training objectives are:

1. The child will discriminate words with /i/ and /u/; for example, *beet* from *boot*.
2. The child will discriminate words with /i/ and /a/; for example, *keep* from *cop*.
3. The child will discriminate words with /u/ and /a/; for example, *coop* from *cop*.
4. The child will identify words with /i/, /u/, and /a/, using a four-item and then six-item response set; for example, *bean* from the response set of: *bean, pot, pit,* and *pool*. The vowels in the response set may include vowels other than /i, u, a/.
5. The child will identify words with /i/, /u/, and /a/ from an open set of familiar vocabulary.

Subsequent training that contrasts other vowels can be incorporated into consonant training activities. Word pairs for meeting Objectives 1, 2, and 3 can be found in Tables 7–2, 7–3, and 7–4, pp. 119, 120, respectively. It is recommended that when the training stimulii are nouns, they be presented in a carrier phrase, such as *That's a _____*. Same/different and Concentration Activities, de-

Table 7–2: Word Pairs That Can Be Used in Achieving the First Vowel Speechreading Training Objective: *The Child Will Discriminate Words with /i/ and /u/.*

beet/boot	mean/moon	she/shoe
he/who	keep/coop	feet/food
speak/spook	heat/hoot	leap/loop
neat/new	teen/tune	see/soup
keep/coop	sheet/shoot	cheap/chew
knee/new	jeep/jewel	*D*/dew
geese/goose	read/root	peel/pool

scribed in Chapter 6, can be used to introduce discrimination and closed-set identification tasks.

consonant speechreading training objectives

Chapter 6 describes three different types of speech features: manner, voice, and place of production. Consonants can be described by these three features (Table 6–7, p. 102). Manner indicates the type of articulatory gestures that are used to produce a sound. For in-

Table 7–3: Word Pairs That Can Be Used in Achieving the Second Vowel Speechreading Training Objective: *The Child Will Discriminate Words With /i/ and /a/.*

heat/hot	keep/cop	need/nod
read/rod	me/mom	pea/pod
seed/sock	heap/hop	cheap/chop
sheep/shop	speak/spot	knee/nod
team/top	jeep/job	see/sod
peak/pop	neat/knot	deal/doll
fear/far	leak/lock	sheet/shot

**Table 7–4:   Word Pairs That Can Be Used in Achieving the
Third Vowel Speechreading Training Objective:** *The Child Will
Discriminate Words with /u/ and /a/.*

new/knot	suit/sock	shoot/shot
coop/cop	food/fox	who/hot
dew/dog	boot/box	moose/moss
loot/lot	room/rot	do/dot
two/top	pool/pot	soup/shop
duel/doll	juice/job	stoop/stop
clue/clock	goose/gone	goose/got

stance, the glide /l/ (*lean*) requires the tongue tip to move downward
in the mouth slowly while the stop /t/ (*teen*) requires it to move quickly.
Glides and stops are two types of manner categories. The other
manner categories are fricatives and affricatives, such as /tʃ/ (*cheap*),
and nasals, such as /m/ (*meat*).

The voicing feature indicates whether or not the consonantal constriction occurs with the vocal cords vibrating. For instance, the pho-
neme /b/ (*bee*) is produced with voice whereas /p/ (*pea*) is produced
without voice.

The place of production feature indicates where in the mouth the
primary constriction for the consonant occurs. For instance, the pho-
neme /b/ (*bass*) has a bilabial place of production (the sound requires
both lips to produce) while /g/ (*gas*) has a velar place of production
(the sound requires the back of the tongue). Other place categories
are labiodental (the sound requires the lower lip and teeth), linguadental (the sound requires the lower lip and teeth), alveolar (the sound
requires the tongue tip), and palatal (the sound requires the center
of the tongue body).

It is fortunate that the visual signal ideally complements the electrical
signal. Cues about manner and voice are easier for implant users to
hear than are cues about place of production. Conversely, cues about
place are easier to see than are cues about manner and voice. For
instance, when an implant user can hear but not see the talker, the

user will likely distinguish between the words *pat* and *bat*. He may not be able to distinguish between *pat* and *cat* using only the auditory signal. On the other hand, the implant user will probably distinguish the word *pat* from *cat* using only the visual signal, but he will not distinguish *pat* from *bat*.

The child should become increasingly reliant on the auditory signal to discriminate consonantal contrasts as he speechreads. Initially, he can be asked to speechread consonants that differ in place of production and that share either manner or voice; for example /p/ as in *pick* and /s/ as in *sick*. The child should quickly experience success since these consonants appear different from one another on the face.

For the next set of discriminations, consonants should share place of production but differ in manner and voice; for example, /p/ as in *pat* and /m/ as in *mat*. These sounds look similar on the face, but they are acoustically different from one another.

Finally, consonants that share both place and manner and/or voice should be practiced; for example, /p/ as in *pat* and /b/ as in *bat*. These sounds will be difficult for the child to distinguish, as they are visually and acoustically similar.

The objectives for consonant speechreading training are:

1. The child will discriminate consonant pairs that differ in place of production and share either voice or manner; for example, *tag* from *bag*.

2. The child will discriminate consonant pairs that share similar place of production but differ in manner and voice; for example, *pan* from *man*.

3. The child will discriminate consonant pairs that share place and manner and/or voice; for example, *park* from *bark*.

4. The child will identify consonants that share manner of production, using a four-item and then a six-item response set; for example, *tag* from the response set of: *tag, bag, back,* and *gas*.

5. The child will identify consonants from a four-item and then a six-item response set of voiced or voiceless consonants; for example, *pop* from the response set of: *pop, cop, cap,* and *top*.

Table 7–5: Consonant and Word Pairs That Can Be Used in Achieving the First Consonant Speechreading Training Objective: *The Child Will Discriminate Consonant Pairs That Differ in Place of Production and Share Either Voice or Manner.*

A. **Consonant pairs**

/m/ (*me*) versus /d/ (*deep*), /dʒ/ (*jeep*), /g/ (*geese*), /j/ (*yeast*), /l/ (*leap*)

/p/ (*pea*) versus /d/ (deep), /tʃ/ (*cheese*), /g/ (*geese*), /ʃ/ (*sheep*), /h/ (*heap*), /s/ (*sea*)

/b/ (*bee*) versus /t/ (*tea*), /dʒ/, /n/ (*knee*), /k/ (*key*), /j/, /l/

/t/ versus /g/, /tʃ/, /θ/ (*thin*)

/d/ versus /k/, /j/, /dʒ/

B. **Word pairs**

meat/geese	peal/heal	bee/tea
nail/jail	tip/chip	bake/cake
pin/chin	map/gap	boat/coat
tie/hi	dog/jog	top/hop
doll/call	bit/knit	pot/hot
tear/chair	pill/chill	moose/goose
pail/sail	make/lake	top/chop

6. The child will identify consonants that share place of production, using a four-item and then a six-item response set; for example, *pan* from the response set of: *pan, man, bat,* and *mat.*

7. The child will identify words from an open set of familiar vocabulary.

Training stimuli for the first three objectives are presented in Tables 7–5, 7–6, 7–7, and 7–8 (pp. 122, 123, 124, 126 and 127). Training stimuli, when nouns, should usually be presented in a carrier phrase context, such as *That's a _____.* Once the child has achieved the objectives above, training can present similar contrasts for consonants in the final position of syllables.

Table 7–6:   Consonant and Word Pairs That Can Be Used for Achieving the Second Consonant Speechreading Training Objective: *The Child Will Discriminate Consonant Pairs That Share Similar Place of Production, but Differ in Manner and Voice.*

A. Consonant pairs

/p/ (*pea*) versus /m/ (*me*), /w/ (*we*)

/d/ (*deep*) versus /s/ (*sea*)

/t/ (*tea*) versus /l/ (*leap*), /n/ (*knee*)

/k/ (*kale*) versus /j/ (*yell*), /dʒ/ (*jail*)

/g/ (*gate*) versus /ʃ/ (*shake*), /tʃ/ (*chain*)

B. Word pairs

pan/man	pea/we	D/see
tail/nail	car/jar	game/chain
cane/Jane	pen/men	pig/wig
dip/sip	tan/land	geese/cheese
day/say	tip/lip	tap/nap
car/yarn	Kim/Jim	girl/shirt
deal/seal	toe/low	take/lake

sentence-level speechreading training objectives

Most children will recognize more speech when they can see and hear than when they can only hear the talker. For this reason, sentence-level speechreading training objectives can begin with more demanding tasks than those for auditory training.

Children will vary greatly in their progress. Some will learn to speechread sentence-level materials rapidly while others will progress slowly. Progress will be influenced by the child's auditory and lipreading skills, how much hearing experience he had prior to receiving an implant, his age at time of implantation, and the effectiveness of the teacher and the appropriateness of the training activities. A child's language and vocabulary skills will greatly influence his progress.

Table 7–7: Consonant and Word Pairs That Can Be Used for Achieving the Third Consonant Speechreading Training Objective: *The Child Will Discriminate Consonant Pairs That Share Place and Manner and/or Voice.*

A. Consonant pairs

/b/ (*bat*) versus /m/ (*mat*), /p/ (*pat*), /w/ (*wet*)

/d/ (*dew*) versus /n/ (*new*), /t/ (*two*), /l/ (*loop*)

/v/ (*vase*) versus /f/ (*face*)

/t/ versus /s/ (*sun*)

/k/ (*K*) versus /g/ (*gay*), /ʃ/ (*shade*), /tʃ/ (*chip*)

B. Word pairs

bat/mat	doll/tall	van/fan
two/Sue	keep/cheek	beak/weak
doe/no	tail/sail	cap/gap
bale/pail	curl/girl	veil/fail
bun/one	dot/knot	toe/sew
cat/gas	dog/log	big/pig
bat/man	kid/chin	tack/sack

Good speechreaders use semantic and syntactic cues to recognize sentences. For instance, most adult speechreaders can guess what the missing word is in the sentence, *The _____ and pepper are on the table.*, even if they are unable to speechread the word *salt*. If the child has limited vocabulary and limited language experience, he will not be able to use such semantic and syntactic cues.

The objectives below require the child to follow simple directions, perform closed-set identification, and listen to topic-related sentences. Ultimately, the child is asked to attend to spoken narratives. The objectives for sentence level training are:

1. The child will follow simple directions using a closed response set.

2. The child will identify a sentence illustration from a set of four dissimilar pictures.

3. The child will identify a sentence illustration from a set of four similar pictures.

4. The child will listen to topic-related sentences, and repeat or paraphrase them.

5. The child will listen to two related sentences, and then draw a picture about them or paraphrase them.

6. The child will speechread a paragraph-long narrative and then answer questions about it.

following directions

Initial exercises can require the child to follow simple instructions with a closed-set of responses; for example, *Color it blue*, where the child has before him three different colors of crayons and a picture of a box.

The response task can become increasingly more difficult as the child's speechreading and language skills improve. For instance, the child might have before him paper and an entire box of crayons. The teacher gives the following instructions, one at a time:

Draw a red house.

Draw a sidewalk by the house.

Draw a bicycle.

Draw a sun in the sky.

Color the sky blue.

closed-set picture identification

The teacher can ask the child to identify a picture illustration from a closed set after he speechreads a simple sentence. For instance, Figure 7–2, p. 128 shows four pictures, a *four-split* response set. For this four-split set, the talker might say, "The woman is cutting the turkey." The child's task is to watch and listen to the talker, and then touch the picture that illustrates the sentence. If the child touches the correct picture, the talker praises him and repeats the sentence a second time. If the child touches the wrong picture, the talker turns the picture face-down or covers it with a piece of construction paper (the same size as the picture). She then says a keyword, "turkey,"

Table 7–8:   Sentences for a Closed-Set Sentence Identification Task (Corresponding to the Four-split Shown in Figure 7–2).

Upper right-hand corner picture
A. The woman is cutting the turkey.

B. The bread is on the counter.

C. The cookies are in the jar.

D. The cookie jar is full.

E. The woman is wearing a dress.

F. The turkey is on the counter.

G. There are two pieces of bread.

H. The woman is standing by the sink.

Upper left-hand corner picture
A. The bicycle tire is flat.

B. The man has a hammer.

C. The man is kneeling.

D. The boy is holding the bicycle.

E. The bicycle is broken.

F. The man and the boy will fix the bicycle.

G. The hammer is in the toolbox.

H. The bicycle is on the ground.

(continued)

and repeats the sentence. This procedure continues until the child selects the correct picture.

Several sentences can be constructed for each picture so that a single four-split set can provide practice for all of them. For instance, the sentences, *The woman is cutting the turkey.* and *The cookies are in the jar.*, can both be spoken for the picture shown in the upper right-hand corner of Figure 7–2. Table 7–8 presents lists of sentences that can be spoken for each of the four pictures shown in this figure.

Table 7–8: *Continued*

Lower right-hand corner picture

A. The man is eating a sandwich.

B. The boy has an apple.

C. The boy is drinking some milk.

D. The boy and the man sit at the table.

E. The boy and the man are eating.

F. The plates are on the table.

G. They are eating lunch.

H. There are two glasses of milk.

Lower right-hand corner picture

A. The children sit on the man's lap.

B. The boy is holding a book.

C. The girl is holding a doll.

D. The man is reading to the children.

E. The man is sitting on the chair.

F. The man is holding the children.

G. The man is reading a story.

H. They are sitting in a big chair.

Pictures from magazines, or snapshots of family members, pets, and friends can be used to construct four-split sets. A teacher might use snapshots taken around the school building. As the child's skills improve, the number of picture options can be increased from four to six. (Tye-Murray [in press] presents additional materials).

One advantage of this activity is that a large number of sentences can be presented in a relatively short period of time. Moreover, it requires the child to speechread for the general idea of a sentence and not necessarily every word, as is the case with a sentence-repetition task. This kind of speechreading resembles a real-world communication task.

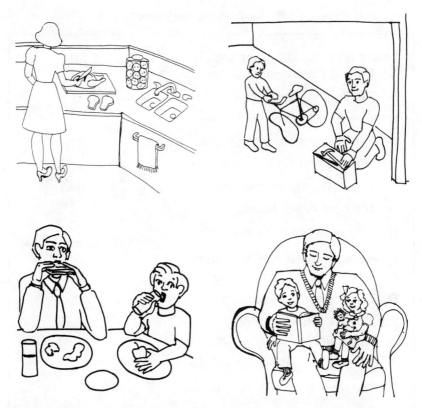

Figure 7–2:   An example of a four-split response illustration for sentence-level speechreading training.

topic-related sentences

Sentences for comprehension activities can center around a common topic. For instance, Tables 7–9, 7–10, 7–11, and 7–12 (pp. 129, 130, 131 and 132) present sentences that a child might hear in a math class, a school library, a school cafeteria, and on the playground. The sentences contain simple vocabulary and syntax. Before speechreading them the child can look at a picture of the setting; for example, a playground. The teacher can describe what the sentences will concern and who might say them. For instance, she might show the child a picture of a girl holding a catcher's mitt and tell him to pretend that he is at recess. She can then say sentences such as, "I caught the baseball.", and "The

Table 7–9:   Math Class Sentences for Topic-related Speechreading Practice.

A. Hand in your homework.

B. We will add the numbers.

C. Come to the blackboard.

D. Work the problems.

E. How much is five plus two?

F. Where is your calculator?

G. Write your name on the paper.

H. Here is a math test.

I. Put your books away.

J. I wrote the number *five*.

K. Write your problem on the board.

L. How many squares?

M. Give me the chalk.

---

bat is by the fence." The advantage of these sentences is that the child practices speechreading vocabulary that he might encounter in a typical school day.

narratives and stories

Lesson objectives can focus on teaching the child to comprehend narratives after he learns to speechread picture descriptions. The teacher might allow the child to look at several pictures about the narrative before she tells the story. This will establish a context for speechreading. She can later ask questions about the story.

conducting a formal lesson

Before the first speechreading session, the child should have his vision checked and, if necessary, receive corrective lenses. If possible, the child should clearly see the talker's face.

**Table 7–10:   Library Sentences for Topic-related
Speechreading Practice.**

A. I want a book about cars.

B. You must be quiet.

C. Sit at this table.

D. The book is on the shelf.

E. I am writing a book report.

F. Where is the pencil sharpener?

G. I found two books.

H. I forgot my glasses.

I. Give me your library card.

J. I will check out this book.

K. Please give me some paper.

L. Have you read this book?

M. Here is my bookbag.

During the initial stages of training, the child must be encouraged to attend to the visual speech signal. Many children who used total communication prior to receiving an implant attend more to the teacher's signs than to her oral movements. Before speaking without sign, the teacher might say, "Look at my face," and point to her mouth. She can talk with and without her lower face visible and ask, "Am I easier to understand when you can watch my mouth?"

Training activities should not distract the child from watching the talker's face. For instance, the child should not look at visual aids, such as an illustration in a book, as the talker speaks.

A variety of stimuli should be used in meeting each of the objectives. If possible, at least five different sets of stimuli should be constructed for each vowel and consonant pair in a discrimination objective. For instance, when the child is to discriminate between /t/ and /b/ (Objective 1 of consonant training), the five sets of word pairs might include, *tag* and *bag, two* and *boo, tall* and *ball, take* and *bake,* and

Table 7–11: Cafeteria Sentences for Topic-related Speechreading Practice.

A. We have hotdogs for lunch.

B. I want some green beans.

C. There are no more forks.

D. Would you like carrots or corn?

E. Take some milk.

F. I need a drinking straw.

G. You dropped your spoon.

H. Do you need a napkin?

I. Please take your lunch tray.

J. I am eating a sandwich.

K. Where is my lunchbox?

L. I want a cookie.

M. Let's sit at this table.

---

tail and *bail*. The child should respond correctly to thirty-five of forty successive presentations before proceeding to a new stimuli pair.

During instruction, the teacher should try to be at the child's eye level at a distance of two to four feet. At this distance, the signal will be loud enough to hear and the child will be able to focus the teacher's face. If a teacher is instructing a group of students, they should sit in a semicircle around her.

The teacher should always use voice when presenting training stimuli and never mouth words. She should speak at a conversational level without exaggerating her articulatory movements.

computer-aided instruction

A few videodisc instructional programs are available for supplementing a speechreading training program (Sims, 1988). A videodisc looks like an audio record and can store about thirty minutes of

**Table 7–12: Recess Sentences for Topic-related
Speechreading Practice.**

A. Will you give me your jump rope?

B. I want to swing.

C. Let's play baseball.

D. I will pitch the ball.

E. Do you have a baseball glove?

F. I want a drink of water.

G. You made a good catch.

H. She hit the ball with a bat.

I. My tennis shoes are new.

J. The bell just rang.

K. I caught the baseball.

L. You hit a home run.

M. Run to first base.

---

audiovisual materials on each side (Figure 7–3). A videodisc is played by a videodisc player, which can be controlled by a computer. Materials stored on a videodisc can be randomly accessed in a short period of time, much like a compact disc.

Tye-Murray, Tyler, Bong and Nares (1988; Tye-Murray, 1991) describe three laser videodisc training programs for hearing-impaired individuals. Students respond to stimuli by touching pictures displayed on a computer touchscreen monitor, so they need not know how to read or type (Figure 7–4, p.134). Program 1 presents words and phrases. Program 2 presents sentences spoken by several talkers, males and females. Program 3 contains related sentences for eleven different settings that a hearing-impaired child might encounter during a typical day; for example, a math class and a school bus. In a typical training exercise, a talker appears on the computer monitor and speaks a sentence. Afterward, four pictures appear on the touchscreen, one of which illustrates the sentence. The child's task is to touch the appropriate illustration.

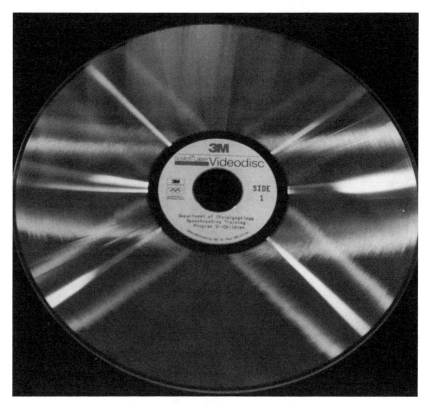

Figure 7–3: A laser videodisc.

Computerized speechreading training will likely become more commonplace as a supplement to teacher-guided instruction. Computerized instruction offers several attractive features. Many training items can be presented in a relatively short period of time, and the computer can maintain a day-to-day record of the child's progress. The child can practice speechreading several different talkers whose speech is stored on a videodisc. To some extent, the child can work independently, thereby removing some demands on the teacher's time.

summary

Children with cochlear implants must develop or re-establish speechreading skills. Initially, formal speechreading training can include phonetic-level and sentence-level objectives. Phonetic-level exercises

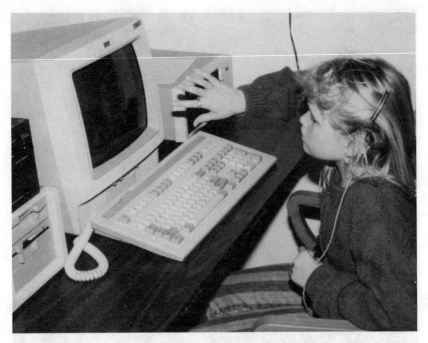

Figure 7–4: An implanted child using a computerized laser videodisc speechreading training program.

should progress in such a way that the child becomes increasingly reliant on the auditory signal for recognizing speech stimuli. As the child's skills develop, speechreading training can include only sentence-level objectives.

references

Jeffers, J., & Barley, M. (1971). *Speechreading (Lipreading)*. Springfield, IL: Charles C Thomas.

Sims, D. (1988). Video methods for speechreading instruction. *Volta Review, 90,* 273–288.

Tye-Murray, N. (1991). Repair strategy usage by hearing-impaired adults and changes following instruction. *Journal of Speech and Hearing Research, 23,* 921–928.

Tye-Murray, N., Tyler, R.S., Bong, B., & Nares, T. (1988). Computerized laser videodisc programs for training speechreading and assertive communication behaviors. *Journal of the Academy of Rehabilitative Audiology, 21,* 143–152.

Tye-Murray, N. (in press). Communication training for hearing-impaired children and teenagers: *Speechreading, Listening and Using Repair Strategies.* Austin, TX: PRO-ED.

Tyler, R.S., Preece, J., & Tye-Murray, N. (1986). *The Iowa Laser Videodisc Sentence Test.* Laser Videodisc, The University of Iowa Hospitals and Clinics.

Walden, B.E., Erdman, S.A., Montgomery, A.A., Schwartz, D.M., & Prosek, R.A. (1981). Some effects of training on speech recognition by hearing-impaired adults. *Journal of Speech and Hearing Research, 24,* 207–216.

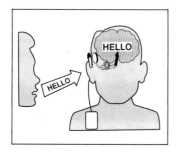

8

communication therapy

nancy tye-murray, ph.d.

An effective listener attends to the talker's message, grasps its important points, and asks the talker to clarify a message when it is misunderstood. Communication therapy teaches hearing-impaired individuals to become good listeners and to use communication strategies (Erber, 1988). Children can learn three communication strategies: a) asking the talker to clarify a misperceived message; b) asking the talker to avoid inappropriate speaking behaviors; and c) correcting or avoiding unfavorable listening environments (Tye-Murray, Purdy, & Woodworth, 1991).

Many children who receive cochlear implants have never learned how to listen and may benefit from communication therapy. Before an implanted child receives communication therapy, however, he must first demonstrate sound awareness and be able to speechread simple sentences. If the child is prelingually deafened, he should have worn his cochlear implant for at least one year. Children over the age of six years are more likely to benefit from therapy than are younger children.

This chapter defines the components of communication therapy and describes training procedures. The components and procedures are presented in the framework of the model shown in Figure 8–1. The

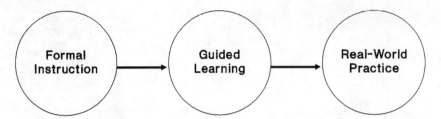

Figure 8–1: A model for teaching implanted children to develop good listening behaviors and to use communication strategies.

model includes: a) formal instruction, b) guided learning, and c) real-world practice. As the child progresses sequentially through these three components, he becomes gradually more proficient in using communication strategies.

formal instruction

Formal instruction introduces good listening behaviors and shows the child how to use communication strategies. This section presents procedures for formally teaching children to listen effectively, to request message clarifications, and to correct inappropriate listening conditions and talker behaviors.

good listening behaviors

Good listening habits are difficult to develop, even for individuals with normal hearing. Elements of good listening behavior are listed in Table 8–1. During formal instruction, a teacher might list the elements on the chalkboard. She can define and demonstrate each one.

Table 8–1: Elements of Good Listening Behavior.

A. Pay attention.
B. Watch the talker's face.
C. Sit up straight.
D. Do not fidget.
E. Identify the talker's main points.
F. Ask questions.

requesting message clarifications

In many instances, a talker may not realize when an implanted child has misunderstood something. In these instances, the child must recognize that he misunderstood the message, alert the talker, and ask for the message to be clarified.

Even when children are using their best listening behaviors, they will often misunderstand spoken messages. They should appreciate this possibility, and learn to detect communication breakdowns. The teacher can draw a talker and a puzzled listener on the chalkboard when defining a communication breakdown. She can then use unfamiliar vocabulary, and ask the children to raise their hands when they do not understand something that she says (Danielle Kelsay, Personal Communication, 1991).

After realizing he has misunderstood a message, the child can request specific information from the talker. This will help the talker better repair the communication breakdown. The symbols in Figures 8–2, 8–3, and 8–4, pp 140–141, show the child what kind of information to request from the talker after a misunderstanding occurs. They include *repeat*, *rephrase*, and *keyword*. The symbols can be photocopied and used during formal instruction. The teacher can point to the *repeat* symbol (Figure 8–2) and say, "When you don't understand a message, ask the talker to say it again." Then she can present examples. She can point to the *rephrase* symbol (Figure 8–3) and say, "You can ask the talker to use different words." The teacher can point to the *keyword* symbol (Figure 8–4) and say, "You can ask the talker to say just one word. This will tell you what the message is about." She can present several examples of rephrased sentences and keywords.

When a communication breakdown has occurred, the talker can best clarify the message when she knows what the child has understood. In the conversation below, the implanted child repeated the part of the message that he recognized:

> **Father:** "We are going to soccer practice after school."
>
> **Chris:** "After school?"
>
> **Father:** "We are going to soccer practice."

When the child repeated what he understood, the father learned explicitly what information was missed. If the child had repeated, "soccer practice", the father might have said, "We are going after school."

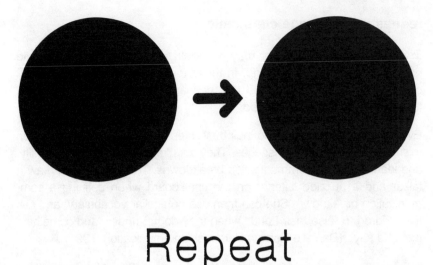

Repeat

Figure 8–2:   An illustration for teaching the *repeat* repair strategy.

A child with adequate speech skills can be encouraged to repeat or rephrase the part of the message that he understands. When the child does not understand a message, the teacher might say, "Tell me what you heard." If the talker knows sign, the child can use total communication if his speech skills are poor.

Most children will experience great difficulty in applying concepts learned during formal instruction to the give-and-take of everyday conversation. Indicating that a communication breakdown has occurred in a gracious and socially acceptable manner can be challenging for even the most accomplished conversationalists. Moreover, finding the words to instruct the talker is not easy. Children will need abundant opportunity to practice repairing communication breakdowns, and teachers should reiterate formally taught concepts many times, in many different contexts.

correcting environmental listening problems and inappropriate talker behaviors

Many individuals who have a long-standing hearing loss realize that poor environmental conditions impair their ability to listen to speech.

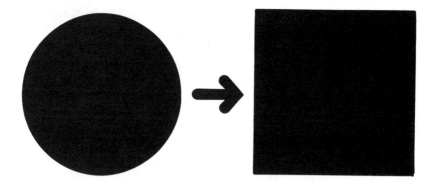

Rephrase

Figure 8–3: An illustration for teaching the *rephrase* repair strategy.

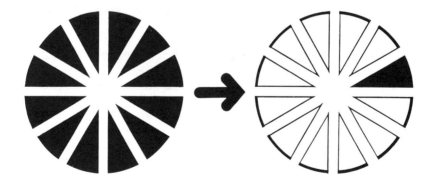

One Word

Figure 8–4: An illustration for teaching the *keyword* repair strategy.

Experience has taught them to correct and even to avoid unfavorable conditions. In contrast, the implanted child may not realize that poor environmental conditions decrease his ability to communicate aurally/orally. He may also not realize that inappropriate talker behaviors affect his ability to speechread, and that he can ask talkers to correct them.

The teacher can write a list of environmental problems and inappropriate talker behaviors on the chalkboard and discuss each one (e.g., Table 8–2). Illustrations such as those shown in Figures 8–5 through 8–16 can be photocopied and used during the discussion. Figure 8–5 shows a boy too far away from the listener. He partially covers his mouth with a book as he speaks. The teacher can point to this picture and ask her students to identify the listening problems. If they are unable to do so, she can ask, "Can you see his mouth? Why not? Is he too far away? What should I tell the boy?" Other speaker and environmental problems are illustrated in Figures 8–6 through 8–16. (See pages 150–160 at the end of this chapter.)

Illustrations such as those shown in Figures 8–17 through 8–24, (see pages 161–168 at the end of this chapter) can be used to teach children how to correct inappropriate talker behaviors. For instance, Figure 8–17 shows an illustration that is captioned, *Don't cover your mouth*. The teacher might photocopy this figure and Figures 8–17 through 8–24 on separate pieces of paper, and place them in a row. She might cover her mouth and say a sentence. Afterward, she can ask with her mouth

Table 8–2:   Environmental Problems That Increase the Difficulty of the Speechreading Task.

A. Poor view of the talker
1. Talker in profile
2. Talker at a distance

B. Poor lighting
1. Light shining in your eyes
2. Talker silhouetted against a light source
3. Talker's face dimly lit

C. Background noise

D. Visual obstructions

E. Visual distractions

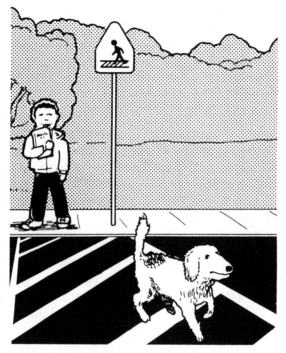

Figure 8–5: An illustration for teaching a child to identify inappropriate talker behaviors: The boy is too far away and he is covering his mouth.

clearly visible, "Why couldn't you understand me? What should you tell me?" The child's task is to select the picture that illustrates her inappropriate talker behavior, and then ask the teacher not to cover her mouth when she speaks.

guided learning

Guided learning focuses the child's attention on good listening behaviors and communication strategies. The child practices the behaviors and strategies in a structured setting. Guided learning has three components: a) modeling, b) role-playing, and c) attention.

modeling

After introducing listening behaviors or communication strategies formally, a teacher can use modeling to demonstrate them. When using modeling, the teacher should explicitly state what is appropriate and inappropriate about the modeled behaviors. She should not assume that the child will recognize this independently. Modeling can be either staged or unstaged. Staged modeling is planned in advance. Unstaged modeling occurs when opportunity arises.

Staged Modeling: During staged modeling, the child might watch the teacher as she demonstrates good and poor listening behaviors. In demonstrating good listening behavior, the teacher sits upright in her chair, watches the talker's face, and avoids unnecessary movements. She raises her hand and asks the talker to clarify a message. In demonstrating poor listening behaviors, the teacher slumps in her chair, does not watch the talker's face steadily, and fidgets with a pencil and a piece of paper. She yawns and looks disinterested. After both models, the teacher points out what was appropriate and inappropriate in her behavior.

In modeling a communication breakdown and subsequent use of a communication strategy, the child's parents might present a staged interaction. For instance, the mother might purposely mumble her speech. The father turns to the child and says, "I didn't understand what she said, did you? I'm going to ask her to say it again." He then asks his wife to repeat her statement.

Unstaged Modeling: In unstaged modeling, the teacher draws attention to good listening behaviors and uses communication strategies.

For instance, the teacher might compliment a student who is paying attention and watching her face.

The teacher might ask for a message clarification when the implanted child is the talker. For example, the child might say, "Swing hit me," and the teacher respond, "Say that in a different way. I didn't understand you." This kind of modeling must be used judiciously. Too many requests for message clarifications, and the child will lose interest in telling a story.

role-playing

A hypothetical listening situation is created during role-playing wherein the child must listen and use communication strategies. When setting up a scene for role-playing, the teacher should select situations that are important to the child; for example, a department store or movie theater. The props should be as realistic as possible so that the child feels as if the interaction was really occurring (Tullos, 1990).

For older children, the teacher might set up a fast-food restaurant, using props such as paper cups, hamburger wrappers, and ketchup packages. The teacher can play the part of employee and the implanted child play the part of customer. The child is assigned the task of ordering dinner for his family. The teacher asks him several questions, such as whether he wants large or small drinks, lettuce on his hamburgers, and so forth. The teacher occasionally speaks with inappropriate behavior, such as speaking in profile. The child must listen to the questions and answer them. When necessary, he must use communication strategies; for example, asking the teacher to look at him when she speaks or asking her to clarify a message.

At the end of the interaction, the child must summarize it. The teacher reviews how effectively he listened and used communication strategies. She might videotape the scenario for more indepth discussion. Other settings for role-playing are listed in Table 8–3.

attention

Teachers and parents can teach children to identify and rectify environmental problems and inappropriate talker behaviors by directing their attention to them. For instance, an implanted child was sitting at the kitchen table. Her mother turned on the faucet and said, "Bring me your dishes." The child did not respond. The mother turned off the water,

Table 8–3:   Situations for Role-playing.

A. Movie theater
   Role of teacher: Concession stand worker
   Child's task: Order popcorn and a drink

B. Shoe store
   Role of teacher: Saleswoman
   Child's task: Buy a pair of tennis shoes

C. Bank
   Role of teacher: Bank clerk
   Child's task: Exchange coins from a piggy bank for dollar bills

D. Library
   Role of teacher: Librarian
   Child's task: Find a book about boats and check it out

E. Department store
   Role of teacher: Saleswoman
   Child's task: Buy a present for a friend's birthday

F. Kitchen
   Role of teacher: Older sibling
   Child's task: Make pancakes

---

pointed to the faucet, and said, "The faucet makes too much noise. I have turned it off. Please bring me your dishes."

In this example, the mother taught the daughter that the faucet is a noise source, a noise source can mask a spoken message, and an unfavorable speechreading environment can be remedied.

real-world practice

Once the implanted child has practiced good listening behaviors in structured settings, he must begin to apply them to his everyday experiences. Real-world practice activities help the child to transfer his listening skills and use of communication strategies to natural settings. Activities should require him to interact with different talkers, in a variety of contexts. Guidelines for developing activities are presented in Table

8–4. This list is adapted from Glennon (1990, pg. 86), who presents guidelines for developing social-skills homework exercises.

The first guideline suggests that the child be able to perform the task successfully during communication therapy before attempting it in a real-world setting. For instance, if the child is to ask the talker to repeat a misperceived message, he should first practice asking for clarification in the classroom. Then the teacher can ask him to attempt the strategy in say, gym class. Although not necessary, the gym teacher can be alerted that the child will practice communication strategies with her.

The next guideline suggests that the child perform the activity in a setting that is meaningful and important to him. For instance, the child might be asked to practice good listening behaviors at a puppet show.

The third guideline for developing real-world practice activities is to select a conversational interaction and setting that will allow the child to experience some success. For instance, in first trying to correct an inappropriate talker behavior, a child will more likely experience success with a normal hearing friend than with a strange clerk in a department store.

The fourth guideline in designing practice activities is to provide written instructions. The instructions should be written with simple vocabulary and sentence structures. For instance, the purpose of a homework activity might be to listen for the main points of a one-paragraph narrative. The classroom teacher would provide the following written instructions, and an envelope:

Table 8–4: Guidelines for Developing Real-world Practice Activities.

A. Assign an activity that the child has performed successfully during communication therapy.

B. Select a setting where the child will feel motivated to communicate.

C. Select an interaction that allows the child to experience some success.

D. Write instructions for the activity, using simple language and vocabulary.

E. Provide a means for the child to record his experience.

> This envelope contains a story. Ask your mother to read it to you. She should
> not use sign. Watch and listen carefully. If you do not understand the story,
> ask questions. Draw a picture about the story.

The final guideline is to provide a means for the child to record his experiences. For instance, in the activity just described, the record is the child's drawing. All students can bring their pictures to class. The teacher can review the story and then ask each child to show his picture. A variation of this activity is to give each child a different story. The child can then show his picture and tell his story. This activity develops both his listening skills and his ability to tell a narrative.

The child can maintain a calendar like that shown in Table 8–5 for one month. The days of the week are listed in a column on the left and people that the child interacts with frequently are listed in a row at the top. The child's task is to record the occasions that he requested a message clarification. During the first week, he is to ask for message repetitions. During the second and third weeks, he is to ask for re-phrasings and keywords, respectively. During the final week, he is to practice repeating or rephrasing what he understood. On every Monday, the teacher reviews the calendar with the child.

summary

Implanted children can learn to use good listening behaviors and communication strategies. They can learn to ask a talker to repeat or re-

Table 8–5: Calendar for Recording Real-world Practice Activity.

When did you ask for a rephrased message?				
	Mom	**Dad**	**Brother**	**Sister**
Monday	at dinner	after school		
Tuesday		before bed		
Wednesday			before school	
Thursday		at soccer practice		
Friday	fixing dinner			before school

phrase a misperceived message, or to repeat a keyword. Children can ensure an optimal listening situation by asking talkers to correct inappropriate speaking behaviors and by correcting or avoiding poor environmental conditions.

Teaching can begin with formal instruction and end with real-world practice. The child should practice good listening behaviors and communication strategies in a variety of communication interactions and in a variety of settings.

references

Erber, N.P. (1988). *Communication Therapy for Hearing-impaired Adults*. Abbotsford, Australia: Clovis Publishing. Alexander Graham Bell Association, Inc.: U.S. Distributor.

Glennon, S.L. (1990). Homework activities for social skills training. In *Teaching Social Skills to Hearing-impaired Students*, P.J. Schloss & M.A. Smith (Eds.), Washington, D.C.: Alexander Graham Bell Association for the Deaf, Inc., 85–90.

Tullos, D.C. (1990). Strategies for assessing and training social skills-facilitator behavior. In *Teaching Social Skills to Hearing-impaired Students*, P.J. Schloss & M.A. Smith (Eds.), Washington, D.C.: Alexander Graham Bell Association for the Deaf, Inc. 45–57.

Tye-Murray, N., Purdy, S., & Woodworth, G. (in press). The reported use of communication strategies by members of SHHH and its relationship to client, talker, and situational variables. *Journal of Speech and Hearing Research*.

Figures 8–6 and 8–7 through 8–24 Mentioned on Page 142.

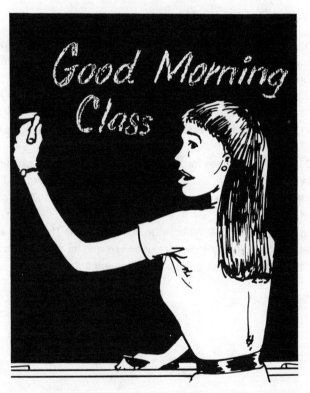

Figure 8–6:   An illustration for teaching a child to identify inappropriate talker behaviors: The teacher is speaking in profile. All of her mouth is not turned towards the listener so that he/she can either hear the sounds or see to lipread.

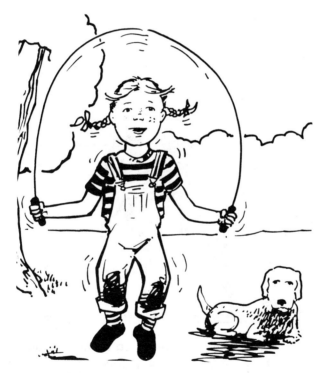

Figure 8–7: An illustration for teaching a child to identify inappropriate talker behaviors: The girl is moving too much.

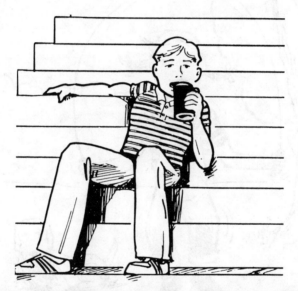

Figure 8–8:   An illustration for teaching a child to identify inap-propriate talker behaviors: The boy is covering his mouth with a soft drink can.

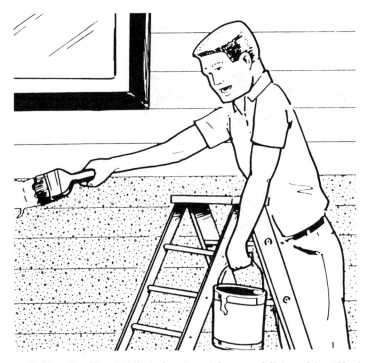

Figure 8–9:   An illustration for teaching a child to identify inappropriate talker behaviors: The man is above the child and is speaking in profile.

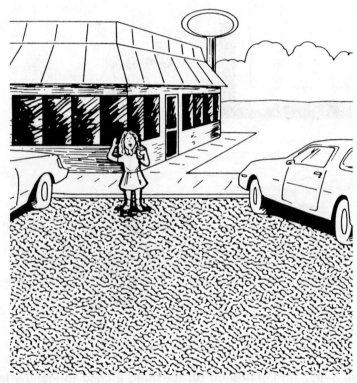

Figure 8–10: **An illustration for teaching a child to identify inappropriate talker behaviors: The girl is too far away either to hear her or to lipread.**

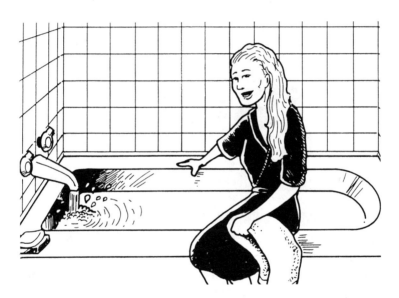

Figure 8–11: An illustration for teaching a child to identify poor environmental conditions: The bath water is running.

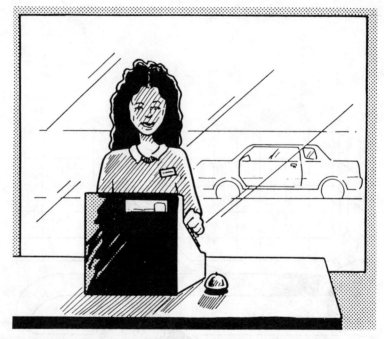

Figure 8–12: An illustration for teaching a child to identify poor environmental conditions: The woman is standing in front of a window. The light is behind her and her face is in the shadow. Also there may be noise from outside.

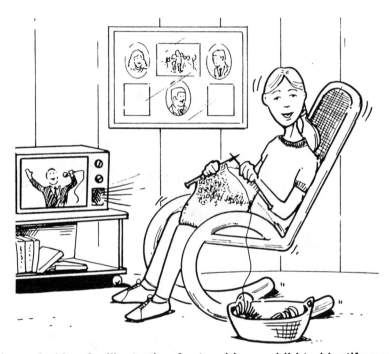

Figure 8–13:   An illustration for teaching a child to identify poor environmental conditions: The television is too loud and the talker is rocking.

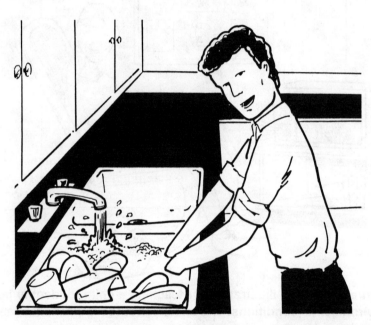

Figure 8–14:   An illustration for teaching a child to identify poor environmental conditions: The water is running.

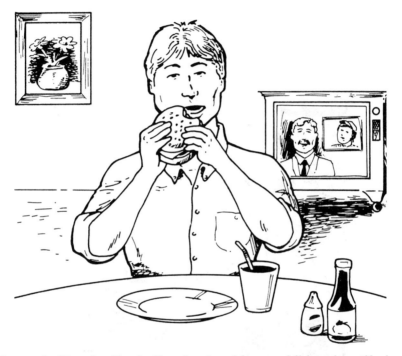

Figure 8–15: An illustration for teaching a child to identify inappropriate talker behaviors and poor environmental conditions: The boy is talking with his mouth full, he is covering his mouth with the sandwich, the television is too loud.

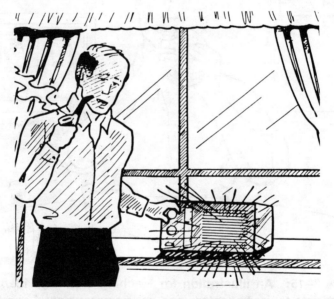

Figure 8–16: An illustration for teaching a child to identify inappropriate talker behaviors and poor environmental conditions: The man is smoking and standing in front of a window, the radio is too loud.

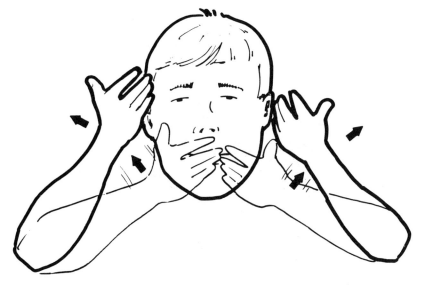

Don't Cover Mouth

Figure 8–17: Illustration for teaching a child to ask someone who is talking not to cover his or her mouth.

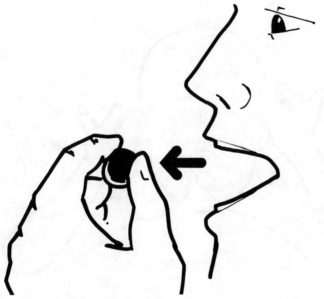

Take Out of Mouth

Figure 8–18: Illustration for teaching a child to ask someone who is talking to remove an object from his or her mouth. The talker should not speak with his/her mouth full.

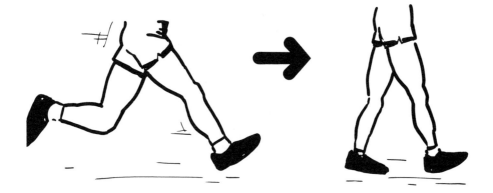

Slow Down

Figure 8–19:   Illustration for teaching a child to ask someone who is talking to slow down his or her speech rate. The concept of a slow speech rate may be difficult for the child to grasp. The teacher might mime a fast versus slow movement, such as jogging or running versus walking in place, and then follow with a demonstration of fast versus slow speech.

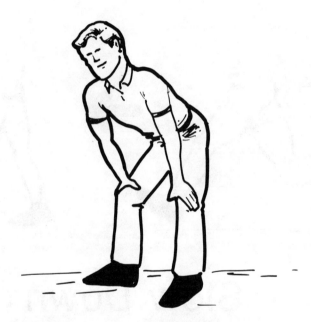

Bend Down

Figure 8–20: Illustration for teaching a child to ask someone who is talking to speak to him at his eye level.

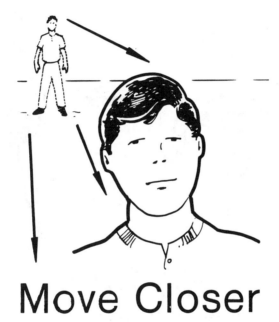

Move Closer

Figure 8–21: Illustration for teaching a child to ask someone who is talking to move closer before speaking.

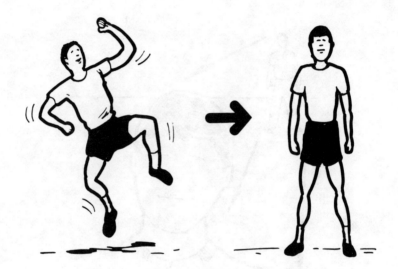

Be Still

Figure 8–22: Illustration for teaching a child to ask someone who is talking to be still and not move while speaking.

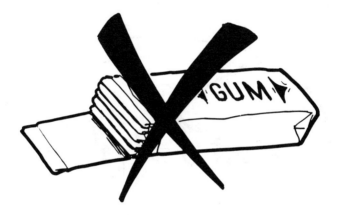

Don't Chew

Figure 8–23: Illustration for teaching a child to ask someone who is talking not to chew gum while speaking.

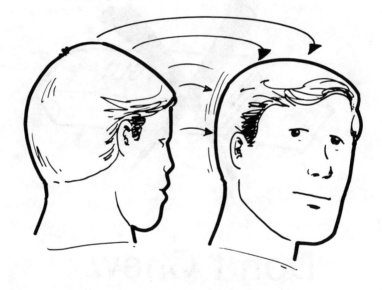

Look at Me

Figure 8–24:   Illustration for teaching a child to ask a talker not to speak in profile.

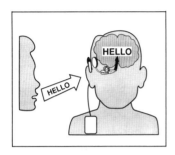

appendix 1—1

troubleshooting the cochlear corporation mini-speech processor

A function check should be completed every day to ensure the implant is in good working condition. This check will take only a few minutes to complete.

function check

1. Turn the control setting on "T" for Test. The "M" (microphone) light on the top of the speech processor should shine continuously. If the child is wearing the implant, he should hear a steady noise. Confirm this.

2. Set the patient controls to user settings. Place the transmitter coil on the side of the speech processor, near the top. The "C" (coil) light should flicker continuously.

3. In a quiet room, hold the microphone approximately one foot from your mouth and say the Ling Five Sounds—/ahh/, /eee/, /ooo/, /sss/, and /shhhh/. The "M" light should flash for each sound. It should not stay on continuously.

If the function check indicates that the implant system is not functioning appropriately, or if your child reports that sound is intermittent or unclear, you must troubleshoot each component to identify the problem.

the speech processor

The speech processor contains the battery which is the power source for the system. If you are using a rechargeable battery, it will probably need to be replaced every day. Regular alkaline batteries will last a little longer than a day. When a battery is dead, remove it immediately.

1. Set the user controls to "T" for test. If the "M" light does not shine continuously, there is a problem with the speech processor. The battery may be dead. If the battery is low, the "M" light will flash slowly. Replace this battery with a new or fully charged one.

2. The battery contacts may be dirty. Clean the silver battery contacts with alcohol on a Q-tip.

3. If the "M" light still does not shine when the processor is set to "T", there may be something wrong with the speech processor. Contact the implant center. If the "M" light shines, but Step 2 of the function check indicates no signal is coming out of the coil, check the cords and the microphone.

the cords

Of all the implant components, the cords are most susceptible to damage. Inspect them once a week to identify breaks in the cord casing which may cause an intermittent signal. Dispose of bad cords once they have been identified.

1. Ensure that the cords are plugged in properly. Match the dot on the cord connecter of the long cord to the dot on the microphone. The end of the cord that plugs into the speech processor will fit in only one way. Check the short cord to ensure each end is plugged in securely to the microphone and the transmitter coil.

2. Replace the long cord that runs from the speech processor to the microphone. Repeat the function check.

3. Replace the short cord that connects the microphone to the coil. Repeat the function check.

4. If step 2 of the function check indicates no signal is coming out of the coil, check the microphone.

the microphone

The microphone can be damaged by moisture, static shocks, and rough handling.

1. If Step 3 of the function check indicates your voice is not being processed, and you have already changed the cords, the microphone may be nonfunctional. You can verify this by trying the hand held microphone which is part of your child's accessory kit. Plug it into the port at the top of the speech processor and repeat Step 3 of the function check. If the hand-held microphone works, but the ear-level microphone does not work, contact the implant center for a replacement of the ear-level microphone.

2. If the microphone has been exposed to moisture, place it in the dri-aid kit immediately. After twelve hours, repeat the function check. If it is still nonfunctional, contact the implant center for a replacement.

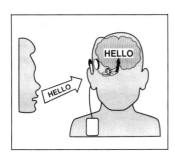

appendix 2·1

coupling an FM system to the cochlear corporation implant (WSP or MSP)

An FM unit can be successfully coupled to the child's cochlear implant if care is taken when setting the controls of the two systems. Because the ear-level microphone of the implant is disengaged when the systems are joined, an FM unit with an environmental microphone is recommended for classroom settings. The child should be evaluated in an audiologic booth in sound field to determine the proper settings for the FM unit and the speech processor.

1. Obtain an appropriate cord from the implant center or from the FM system manufacturer to couple the child's FM receiver to the speech processor. This cord connects the audio output or headphone jack of the receiver to the input port on the top of the speech processor.

2. Ensure that the FM system and the cochlear implant system are functioning properly before attempting to join the two. Complete an electroacoustic analysis and a listening check of the FM

system, evaluating separately the teacher microphone and the environmental microphone as a sound source. Complete a function check of the cochlear implant system (Table 2–1, p. 28). Obtain a sound field audiogram of the child's threshold responses to speech and to warble tones across frequencies with the implant alone.

3. Set the frequency response and the output controls of the FM unit to a flat, broad response with an output of approximately 30 dB SPL. The output control may have to be adjusted to provide more or less gain depending on the child's responses when the speech processor and FM systems are turned on (see Steps 7–9).

4. With the FM system and the speech processor **turned off**, plug in the connecting cord between them. Place the child's transmitter coil and microphone on his ear as usual and set the speech processor to **N** and the sensitivity control to **0**.

5. The teacher microphone and the environmental microphone on the child's FM receiver must be evaluated individually. First, **turn on the volume control of the child's receiver to the minimum setting**. Turn off the environmental microphone and turn on the teacher microphone and the child's receiver.

6. Talking into the teacher microphone, slowly turn up the child's speech processor to his typical user setting. Once at user setting, slowly increase the volume on the child's receiver from the minimum setting to a comfortable listening level.

7. Evaluate the child in the sound field with the teacher microphone placed at a calibrated distance from the speaker. Adjust the volume control of the child's receiver and check his responses in sound field until you obtain warble tone thresholds and a speech detection threshold similar to the child's responses with the implant alone. It may be necessary to adjust the gain control of the receiver or the user settings of the speech processor to achieve the desired response. WSP users often must use a speech processor setting of **1**. Record these settings.

8. Turn the receiver volume control to the minimum setting. Turn off the teacher microphone and turn on the environmental microphone of the receiver. The speech processor should be on user settings. Talking into the environmental microphone, increase the volume on the child's receiver to a comfortable listening level.

9. Repeat Step 7 but instead of using the teacher microphone, place the child wearing the receiver at a calibrated distance from the speaker. In completing Steps 7 though 9, do not set the volume control of the FM receiver or the sensitivity control of the speech processor at the highest setting. Instead increase the output gain of the receiver if needed.

10. Using the settings you have obtained in the previous steps, ask the child about the sound quality using the FM unit compared to using the implant alone. It may be appropriate to compare the two conditions using auditory discrimination tasks.

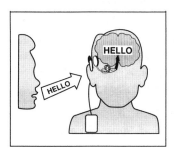

appendix 2-2

auditory training tests and materials

A. *The Developmental Approach to Successful Listening* (DASL), 1986. Gayle Goldberg Stout and Jill Van Ert Windle.

Available from: DASL, Ltd.
726 Diamond Leaf
Houston, TX 77079

The DASL is an easy to use curriculum guide that focuses on the hierarchical development of auditory skills. It includes a placement test, illustrations for therapy activities, a list of resources, and checklists to assist in defining therapy goals.

B. *Early Speech Perception Test for Profoundly Hearing-Impaired Children* (ESP), 1990. Ann Gears and Jean Moog.

Available from: Central Institute for the Deaf
818 South Euclid Avenue
St. Louis, MO 63110

The ESP is a battery of tests that can be used to establish objectives for and to measure the effectiveness of auditory training. The ESP includes a special battery of low verbal tests that can be used with children as young as two to three years old who have limited verbal abilities.

C. *Test of Auditory Comprehension* (TAC), 1981. Los Angeles County Schools.

> Available from: Foreworks
> Box 9747
> North Hollywood, CA 91609

The TAC consists of audio-taped subtests of auditory skills ranging from simple discrimination to comprehension and auditory memory tasks. It is one component of the Auditory Skills Instructional Planning System. The other components are the Auditory Skills Curriculum Guide and the Audio Worksheets which include specific activities and materials for auditory training.

D. *Communication Training for Hearing-Impaired Children and Teenagers: Speechreading, Listening and Using Repair Strategies.* In press. Nancy Tye-Murray.

> Available from: PRO-ED
> 8700 Shoal Creek Boulevard
> Austin, TX 78758-6897

These materials provide auditory and speechreading training, and provide practice in using verbal strategies to repair communication breakdowns. The language and vocabulary are relevant to students' everyday activities.

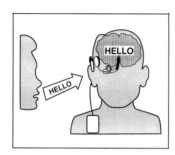

appendix 2·3

speech and language tests for hearing-impaired children

a. speech tests

Phonetic Level Speech Evaluation, in Ling, D. *Speech and the Hearing-Impaired Child: Theory and Practice*, 1976.

    Available from: Alexander Graham Bell
                      Association for the
                      Deaf, Inc., 1976.
                      3417 Volta Place, N.W.
                      Washington, D.C. 20007

    This evaluation assesses the child's ability to imitate the non-segmental and segmental aspects of speech. Order of item presentation follows the natural hierarchy of speech development. The automaticity of production is evaluated by requiring the child to repeat the target sounds in increasingly complex phonetic environmental sounds.

Phonologic Level Speech Evaluation, in Ling, D. *Speech and the Hearing-Impaired Child: Theory and Practice*, 1976.

Available from: Alexander Graham Bell
                 Association for the
                 Deaf, Inc., 1976.
                 3417 Volta Place, N.W.
                 Washington, D.C. 20007
This test evaluates the degree to which nonsegmental and segmental speech patterns have become part of the child's linguistic repertoire.

Levitt, H., Youdelman, K., and Head, J. *Fundamental Speech Skills Test* (FSST), 1990.
        Available from: Resource Point, Inc.
                         61 Inverness Dr. East
                         Englewood, CO 80112
This test assesses the breath stream management, underlying articulatory coordination, pitch control, phrase production, and spontaneous speech. Specific guidelines for scoring the nonsegmental and segmental aspects of speech are provided.

Monsen, R. *SPeech INtelligibility Evaluation* (SPINE), 1981.
        Available from: Publications Office
                         Central Institute for the Deaf
                         818 South Euclid
                         St. Louis, MO 63110
This test is intended as a measure of intelligibility for severely and profoundly hearing-impaired adolescents.
The SPINE consists of sets of phonemically contrasting words that the child reads. Results are expressed as the number of words correctly understood by the examiner.

Monsen, R., Moog, J., and Geers, A. *Picture SPINE* (SPeech INtelligibility Evaluation), 1988.
        Available from: Publications Office
                         Central Institute for the Deaf
                         818 South Euclid
                         St. Louis, MO 63110
The Picture SPINE is intended to provide a measure of speech intelligibility for severely and profoundly hearing-impaired children. The test is organized into sets of pictures that the child names. Results are expressed as a percentage of words correctly identified by the examiner.

b. language tests

Moog, J.S., and Geers, A.S. *Grammatical Analysis of Elicited Language—Pre-Sentence Level* (GAEL-P), 1983.
Available from: Publications Office
Central Institute for the Deaf
818 South Euclid
St. Louis, MO 63110
This test uses a set of fifty objects to evaluate the receptive and expressive language skills of severely and profoundly hearing-impaired children. Normative data for hearing-impaired children aged three to six years are provided.

Moog, J.S., and Geers, A.S. *Grammatical Analysis of Elicited Language—Simple Sentence Level* (GAEL-S), 1979.
Available from: Publications Office
Central Institute for the Deaf
818 South Euclid
St. Louis, MO 63110
This test uses toy manipulation to evaluate the receptive and expressive language skills of severely and profoundly hearing-impaired children. Normative data are provided for hearing-impaired children aged four to ten years, and for normal-hearing children aged two and a half to five years.

Moog, J.S., and Geers, A.S. *Grammatical Analysis of Elicited Language—Complex Sentence Level* (GAEL-P), 1980.
Available from: Publications Office
Central Institute for the Deaf
818 South Euclid
St. Louis, MO 63110
This test uses toy manipulation to evaluate the receptive and expressive language skills of severely and profoundly hearing-impaired children. Normative data are provided for hearing-impaired children aged eight to twelve years, and for normal-hearing children aged three to six years.

Engen, E., and Engen, T. *Rhode Island Test of Language Structure* (RITL), 1983.
Available from: PRO-ED
8700 Shoal Creek Boulevard
Austin, TX 78758-6897

This test is designed to assess receptive language skills. Stimulus sentences are presented by the examiner, and the child indicates the appropriate sentences by choosing among three pictures. A range of simple sentence structures are examined. Normative data are presented for normal-hearing children aged three and a half to six years, and for hearing-impaired children aged five to seventeen years.

Quigley, S.P., Steinkamp, M.W., Power, D.J., and Jones, B.W. *Test of Syntactic Abilities*, 1978.
Available from: Dormac, Inc.
P. O. Box 752
Beaverton, OR 97075

This test was constructed to measure comprehension and use of English syntactic structures. It includes a screening test and twenty individual diagnostic tests. The ability to read and write is required. Normative data for profoundly, prelingually hearing-impaired students aged ten years to eighteen years, eleven months are provided.

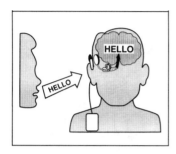

appendix 6·1

auditory training activities for parents to perform with their newly implanted child

A pamphlet provided to parents at the University of Iowa Hospitals and Clinics.

awareness

The first level of auditory development is sound detection or awareness. Awareness activities are described in this section.

listening walk

Sound through the implant may initially have no meaning for your child. You must help him associate meaning with the sounds that he hears. Take a *listening walk*. Identify the presence of sound in the environment. Close doors, run water, flush toilets, play with noisemaking toys. Go outside and identify sounds. Walk around the neighborhood. Nearly everything we do involves some kind of noise. The child will need to be alerted to the presence of sound at first. He will have to learn, or possibly relearn, to interpret sounds in his environment. Always locate the source of sound, and, if appropriate, provide a sign to signify its meaning.

peek-a-boo

Teaching a child to respond to his name is a goal that all parents have for their implanted child. Achieving this goal may take several weeks or months. A peek-a-boo activity will begin the training process. Tell your child to listen for his name. Ask him to cover his eyes or turn him around with his back toward you. Say his name loudly and give him a cue that you have done so by either tapping his shoulder or by turning him around. After he understands the game, try again without the cue. If he is successful, praise him generously! It may be fun to turn the tables and ask him to say your name while you wait with covered eyes. Once the child responds correctly 100 percent of the time, practice this skill during other activities; for example, while he works on a puzzle. Instruct him that before the puzzle is finished, you will call his name and he should look up.

volume control

We all like to control our environment. The child can perform and enjoy a *volume control* activity. Allow him to play with a small radio or tape player. Show him the volume control and demonstrate *soft* and *loud*. Indicate when the sound is too loud or too soft. Give the child the radio and encourage him to change the volume. (The next lesson the child may need to learn is when this activity is allowed.) Noise-making toys that the child can play with independently also develop sound aware-ness skills.

musical chairs

Your child can finally play this game and not be the first one "out". Use a tape recorder or record player. Instruct your child to march around the floor as long as he hears music. When the music ends, he sits down. This activity can also be done using a musical instrument, a hair dryer, or other noise-making machine. Keep the task from becoming boring by changing the child's required response. For example, the child can stack blocks or color until the sound stops.

sound discrimination

Once your child can reliably detect sound, he can begin to discriminate environmental sounds and speech. For formal teaching, start with a limited set of two or three sounds; for example, the phrases, *Hi!* and *See you later!*. In this example, you might say one of the phrases and your child will move a doll toward or away from you as appropriate. For informal training, talk about how one sound differs from another; for example, the telephone has an on/off pattern, the dishwasher makes a continuous sound, the microwave makes three short beeps, and so forth.

let's make some noise

Find several small objects that make different noises; for example, a set of keys, a small whistle, a drum, a small bell. Use only two of the objects at a time. First, make a noise with the object while the child watches and listens. Ask him to name the object. Repeat the activity without showing him the noise-maker. In the bathroom, use the hair dryer, the toilet flushing, and the water faucet as noise-makers. In the kitchen, operate an electric can opener, shake a box of cereal, and clang some pots.

voiced patterns

Using voice, speak a pattern and offer the two response choices to the child, using either pictures, toys, or signs as response choices. Take turns: these kinds of activities also develop the child's speech skills. Example speech patterns are:

> **Short versus long sound;** for example, sustained *ahhh* versus *ahhhhhhhhh.*

> **Continuous versus interupted sounds;** for example, sustained *ahhhh* versus *ah ah ah ah ah ah ah ah.*

> **One versus two sounds;** for example, ba versus ba ba.

> **Slow versus fast sounds;** for example, *ba . . . ba . . . ba . . .* versus *babababababa.*

> **Soft versus loud sound.**

These speech patterns can be practiced using objects or toys, as described below:

(short versus long)	*The car goes beep and the cow says moooooooooooooo.*
(continuous versus interrupted)	*The whistle goes eeeeeeee and the drum goes boom boom boom.*
(one versus two)	*The dog says woof and the cat says meee-owww.*
(slow versus fast)	*This car is slow and goes putt . . . putt . . . putt.*
	This car is fast and goes puttputtputtputt.
(loud versus soft)	*The keys make a loud jangle and the bear makes a soft squeak.*

speech discrimination

The most important and useful sound the child will hear is speech. When the implanted child realizes that sound is meaningful and can aid communication, he has reached a milestone. He may increasingly depend on the auditory signal for information. The following activities will help nurture this development.

vocabulary games

Ask the child to discriminate simple words. Remember that discrimination implies choosing from a closed set. Work with different categories of items, such as family names, colors, shapes, or animals using pictures, cut-out shapes, or toys that represent each word in the set. Place the alternatives before the child. Initially, response sets should contain words or phrases that vary in length or in syllable number. The child may not have developed the ability to discriminate words that are similar in length and phonetic composition; that may take many months of experience. Examples of response sets that can be used for discrimination activities include:

    a. **Family names or household pets;** for example, *Mommy* versus *Tim*, *kitty cat* versus *dog*.

    b. **Colors;** for example, *yellow* versus *red*, *blue* versus *purple*.

c. **Shapes;** for example, *triangle* versus *star*, *rectangle* versus *oval*.

d. **Animals;** for example, *dog* versus *elephant*, *cat* versus *alligator*, *rabbit* versus *pig*.

Combine colors, shapes or items for a longer and more difficult discrimination task or ask the child to manipulate the toys; for example:

Find a green circle (or a red square).

Show me the green banana (or the red strawberry).

Where is the pink elephant (or the blue bear)?

Put the man on the horse. (Move the red car.)

If the activities are too difficult to perform using only the auditory signal, allow your child to speechread you. As a general rule, discrimination activities should start with words, phrases or sentences that are very different in length or syllable number. As the child's auditory discrimination abilities improve, use more challenging items that are similar in length.

"go fish," and other commercially-available games

Commercially-available games that require the participants to request something of one another or announce the next move require speech production and listening skills. Contextual cues are often high and the number of response alternatives is limited. For instance, in the game *Go Fish* the child has to listen to the other players' requests in order to participate. In board games, such as *Candyland*, the child's opponent can read the cards that dictate activities. The child must listen (or speechread) to know his next move. Explore the games that interest your child, and modify them to include speech production and listening activities.

"i see something" . . . , and other guessing games

Most children like games that require some imagination. *I see something* is a game that the implanted child can play with parents, sibling or friends in several different environments. Colors or descriptors can be used, for example, *I see something red . . . I see something fuzzy . . . I see something you use to clean things . . . .* The contextual cues are high and alternatives are limited. Take turns listening and speaking. Encourage the child to use his speech. Part of the challenge for the child's playmate can be determining what cue was given by the implanted child.

Guessing hidden objects will be more difficult and may be appropriate for an older child. Put a small object in a paper bag and take turns asking questions and making guesses about the object's identity. Use a predetermined set of objects to limit the possible questions. For example, put the following objects on the table: scissors, an apple, a paper clip, a piece of candy, a pencil, a stick of gum, an eraser, a marble, and a toy car. Have the child put one of the items in the bag, without showing you which one. Ask him questions about the object until you are able to guess its identity; for example, *Is it red?*, *Can you eat it?*.

speech comprehension

When your child can detect and discriminate a sound or spoken message, associate meaning to that signal, and then respond appropriately, he has reached a level of auditory development known as comprehension. Comprehension skills evolve naturally as a child learns to use sound in a meaningful way. However, these skills may need to be nurtured and encouraged with training activities.

A child may demonstrate auditory comprehension of environmental sounds by picking up the telephone when it rings, opening the door of the microwave when it beeps, or quieting a dog when it barks. Comprehension of speech is the most difficult and sophisticated speech task.

An implanted child demonstrates comprehension of speech when he responds to his name, follows directions, or responds to questions. Often situational or an environmental context helps the child to comprehend a spoken message. For example, in a daily routine such as eating breakfast, a child who answers appropriately when asked orally what kind of cereal he wants, has demonstrated auditory comprehension. As auditory comprehension skills develop, parents may observe their child using less sign language and relying more on speechreading and listening: encourage these behaviors. Occasionally omit signs when talking to your child, as when asking him to set the table or clean his room.

The development of auditory skills varies greatly among implanted children. It is not possible to predict how long it will take for a child to master the skills described above. However, we have found two factors that foster development. First, children who quickly accept the implant and begin wearing it all waking hours appear to develop auditory skills faster than those who use the implant only occasionally. Secondly, listening practice in the home and support from parents and other family members appear to accelerate successful development.